Luiz Eduardo Almeida
Marília Nalon Pereira

Oral health

Luiz Eduardo Almeida
Marília Nalon Pereira

Oral health

A question of education

ScienciaScripts

Cover image: www.ingimage.com

This book is a translation from the original published under ISBN 978-3-330-76835-2.

Publisher:
Sciencia Scripts
is a trademark of
Dodo Books Indian Ocean Ltd. and OmniScriptum S.R.L publishing group

120 High Road, East Finchley, London, N2 9ED, United Kingdom
Str. Armeneasca 28/1, office 1, Chisinau MD-2012, Republic of Moldova, Europe
Managing Directors: Ieva Konstantinova, Victoria Ursu
info@omniscriptum.com

Printed at: see last page
ISBN: 978-620-8-59582-1

Summary

Authors

Luiz Eduardo de Almeida

Graduated in Dentistry from the Federal University of Juiz de Fora (UFJF/2007), specialist in Collective Health (UFJF/2008) and master's degree in Clinical Dentistry/Collective Health (UFJF/2010). He is an Assistant Professor in the Department of Dentistry at the Governador Valadares Advanced Campus of the Federal University of Juiz de Fora, working in teaching, research, extension and management. The following areas of activity are described: Health Sciences (Major Field), Dentistry (Field of Knowledge), Social and Preventive Dentistry (Subfield) and Collective Health (Specialty).

Marilia Nalon Pereira

Graduated in Dentistry from the Federal University of Juiz de Fora (1977), resident/specialist in Oral and Maxillofacial Surgery from the Fluminense Federal University (1982-1984), Master in Fundamentals of Education from the Juiz de Fora Higher Education Center (2000), PhD in Restorative Dentistry from the São Paulo State University Júlio de Mesquita Filho (2002) and Specialist in Public Health from the Federal University of Juiz de Fora (2004). Associate Professor III at the Federal University of Juiz de Fora. She has experience in Dentistry, with an emphasis on Clinical Dentistry, working mainly on the following subjects: surgery, dentistry, prevention, education and health promotion.

Almeida, Luiz Eduardo de; Pereira, Marilia Nalon. Oral health: a question of education / Luiz Eduardo de Almeida. Novas Edições Acadêmicas. 2017. 157f.

Supervisor: Prof[a] Dr[a] Marilia Nalon Pereira Monografia (graduação) - Faculty of Dentistry - UFJF ORE Department, Faculty of Dentistry, 2007

1. Health. 2. Education. 3. psychomotricity. Monograph. I. Faculty of Dentistry, Federal University of Juiz de Fora. ORE Department, Dentistry. II. Pereira, Marilia Nalon (Supervisor). III. Oral health: a question of education.

Dedication

I dedicate this work, first and foremost, to my worthy parents, Celso (In memori an) and Gracinha - people of integrity and true examples of life and character. I owe my life, my moral formation and my achievements to them.

I also offer it to my siblings, Adriana, Celso, Ronaldo, Pedro and Luciana, of whom I am so proud. I also leave here the names of my beloved nephews: Graziele, Pablo, Matheus, Gustavo, Ana Carolina, Lucas and Luisa.

I couldn't fail to mention my dear uncles, Joaquim, Marcos and Jorge, who were instrumental in making my dream come true: graduating in dentistry.

Know that together you are the truest meaning of the words love and friendship. I love you!

Luiz Eduardo de Almeida

Thanks

There are certainly many examples to follow. I think that giving thanks is not just remembering a few names or places, but recognizing the importance they have had in my life.

Therefore, I would like to thank the Faculty of Dentistry, the Professors, the Staff and my Friends who accompanied me throughout the course. Thus, remembering definitive personalities is not enough in view of the importance they had at this stage of my life. Please know that you have brought a special meaning to my way of life.

Thank you for being there and for being part of my story.

Luiz Eduardo de Almeida

"The value of things is not in how long they last,

but in the intensity with which they happen.

That's why there are unforgettable moments,

inexplicable things

and incomparable people"

Fernando Pessoa

Preface

The aim of this study is to describe a model of comprehensive health care, discarding the care model, which is centered on the disease and based on care for those who seek it.

As far as oral health is concerned, it is known that caries and periodontal diseases still affect many people. With a view to halting, regressing and, above all, preventing these diseases, a motivational project will be described here, the methodology of which is based on HEALTH EDUCATION, with a view to learning and apprehension, as well as turning learners into carriers of knowledge.

There will be 16 stages: Introduction, Good manners, My home, My family, Habits and notions of hygiene, Sense organs, Food and nutrition, Preventing domestic accidents, Dentists and doctors are our friends, Teeth and their functions, Caries and periodontal disease, Toothbrushing, Toothpaste and Floss, Brushing my teeth, Plaque remover and Floss, Closing. All the stages will include fun activities that will explore psychomotor skills during the school year.

In this way, as well as working on health-related issues, leisure will also be provided for those who receive care, in other words, a combination of learning and pleasure. Thus, in this line of research qualification, still related to its aims, it is concluded that it is not possible to separate the attitudes and procedures of care aimed at education, from the attitudes and procedures aimed at promoting health, just as it is not possible to separate the biological, the social and the psycho-affective.

1. introduction

The great discoveries began with doubt, questioning, or rather, questions, and so they came to fruition - just go back in history and see how they came about.

Today's world provides us with a lot of information - television, books, the internet, magazines, conferences and newspapers - which confuses people because they don't know what questions to answer. We have a generation that is obsessed with answers, but has difficulty asking questions. Individuals accumulate data, but have difficulty applying it. According to Alves (2005), p.16, "*Thinking is knowing how to ask questions*". He also states that "*Our intelligence developed to compensate for our bodily incompetence*".

So where are the valuable questions? And why are so many answers being sought? Nothing replaces the pleasure of discovery, even when it comes to things that have already been discovered. An example of this is children, who know the world of questions and who, unfortunately, are often castrated by adults and even by the educational institution itself, when in fact the latter should learn from them. Asking questions is the basis of education.

So this work began with a question: what is more important to know, about health or about illness? Before you continue reading, think about it. Of course, if most, if not all, people were asked this question, they would answer that health outweighs illness in terms of importance. However, when you think about it, you can clearly see a contradiction between the above answer and the reality that follows. If health were really so important and valued, why are people so sick? There is talk of the genome, cloning, transplants, the latest generation of drugs, miracle vaccines, in other words, with each passing day the "advances" in medical science become clear, and in contrast to all this, more diseases are appearing, and even returning. In fact, Maranhâo (2000) states that illness is becoming something common, expected, a natural attribute. Is science heading in the right direction? And if not, what is the reason for so many failures? According to Rossetti (1999), p. 77, "You don't have to adapt patients to science, you have to adapt science to people", in other words, when you manage to reconcile science and humanization, you will arrive at the much sought-after health.

It normally takes a dentist an average of five years to graduate. During the course of the dentistry course, students attend courses designed to teach them how to diagnose and treat the diseases that affect the complex oral cavity; in other words, in the university environment itself, disease is given pride of place. In practical courses, the sicker the patient, the better, and academics even discuss: "I took a patient who has everything to do", or even worse, "I wasn't lucky today, my patient had nothing, I sent him away". In this last case, it is curious that the academic, and often the teacher himself, is not prepared to work with health, since a treatment plan should be drawn up for this patient to preserve his oral health, so that he doesn't come back sick after a while. In fact, according to Brasil (1998), the patient should not be discharged, but the disease. Why do health professionals feel responsible only for the illness and not for health? Isn't this appreciation of the disease responsible for the frequent fear that some patients feel towards doctors and dentists? Sometimes this is because they believe they will find disease there and never health. However, it is important that health programs consider the demystification of illness as a fatality or something inevitable, or even irrelevant to general well-being (ALONSO, 1990; BATISTA, 2006; FERREIRA et al., 2004; ROSSETTI, 1999).

According to Ainamo (1989), Carvalho and Maltz (1999), Chiapinotto (2000) and Torriani (1996), with regard to **oral health**, it can be said that, in many populations, practically all individuals have or have had experience with dental caries or periodontal disease, or even both. In fact, as cited by Maranhâo (2000), it can be said that these diseases are often not even considered as such, in other words, they are becoming normal. For Ainamo (1989), Carvalho and Maltz (1999), Chiapinotto (2000) and Torriani (1996), there is no doubt that for them to occur, plaque must be deposited. Alves et al. (2003), p. 192, stated that *"the combination of toothbrush and dental floss, when used correctly, are the main factors responsible for the mechanical removal of bacterial biofilm"* - preventive methods that are easy to access. But despite the fact that these diseases are widely known and simple to prevent, why has dentistry, with its extensive technical and scientific apparatus, still not managed to stop them, or at least reduce their high rates? Simple, because the current teaching model offered at dental schools, the biomedical model, is incapable of providing health care for a large part of the population, since it does not focus on collective health. According to Amaral (1991), university training is very deficient in relation to subjects that deal with social and preventive aspects, leading in many cases to a lack of interest on the part of future professionals. Harrison (2003) in his studies mentions that universities should take on the role of reflecting on what they are producing and reproducing, since these institutions have a direct commitment to the health of society.

An interesting example: an individual - no need to ask about gender, age, race and the like - makes an appointment with a dental surgeon. During the appointment, the dentist usually asks the patient to open his mouth for further assessment. Imagine that this patient has 28 teeth and that only four of them have carious lesions. What often happens? The professional would take out a piece of paper, sketch out a budget and then tell the patient that they have caries and that treating the diseased teeth would cost a certain amount. Frustrating, but it's the reality - we are currently living in the commercialization of health, indeed of disease, and the massacre of humanized care.

Returning to the last case mentioned, the dentist focused only on the diseased teeth. What about the other 24 healthy teeth? At any point during the consultation was it explained to the patient that tooth decay is a highly mutilating infectious disease which, fortunately, can be controlled, treated and, above all, prevented? No. In fact, it's rare for professionals to do so - dentists forget that they have the role of educators, i.e. it's not just about making a resin or amalgam restoration, for example, but also about educating their patients to receive them when necessary. As a result, men usually reach old age without teeth, something they think is natural. Rossetti (1999), p.16, asks: *"Why do human beings have dentistry, which is supposed to protect them, and they don't have teeth; animals, which don't have dentistry, preserve their teeth"*.

As stated by Brasil (1998), Cadernos de Educaçao Popular 7 (1984) and Herzlich (1991), health professionals often "treat" their patients by starting with the disease in order to achieve health. Why not turn this around? We would have a service that values health and not illness.

With regard to preventive methods, despite the fact that they are cheap, effective and usually simple to apply - as mentioned by Brasil (1998), WHO (1998) and Rouquayrol (1993) - why is there so much reluctance, or even prejudice, in using them? Or rather, what is lacking to get these mechanisms applied, adopted and, above all, accepted by the population? Is this not a problem of education? Are dentists only being educated to cure disease? Or are they able to educate their patients about their state of oral health, the treatment proposed to them and, above all, how to maintain their health? Who is wrong, the dentist or the patient? In fact, everyone is wrong. The professionals, who are being educated to "cure" diseases, and the patients are wrong because they are not interested in their own health, as Rossetti (1999), p.19, states:

"Dentists are not entirely to blame. Man has changed the way he eats, his habits, he has started to use a fork and knife, he has cooked food, he has incorporated sugar into his diet. So the first thing to blame is man himself. Primitive man had a different way of behaving, which allowed him to rely on self-cleaning."

The purpose of this paper is to describe a different way of working in health, through education, in other words, **health education**. Ideas will be offered here, not techniques to be copied or imitated; in fact, from conversations, meetings and discussions, solutions can emerge.

It's not just for dentists, but for teachers, community leaders, parents and, above all, for those who want to make their health essential. After all, taking care of your own health is within everyone's reach and is not a task to be delegated only to professionals. In fact, health is created and lived on the edge of everyday life: in the centers of education, work and leisure. According to Brasil (1998), Cadernos de Educaçao Popular 7 (1984), Conselho Regional de Nutricionistas (2006), Matos (1998), Minayo et al (2000), WHO (1998), Pettry et al (1997), Rufino Netto (1994), health is not a disease, health is quality of life.

2. Theoretical background

2.1 Health education

The word health has taken on very diverse and even contradictory meanings. According to Brasil (1998), the fact is that health and illness do not designate abstract values or absolute situations, nor are they static conditions - obviously change, and not stability, is predominant in life, both from an individual and social point of view.

Therefore, in order to characterize health, according to Valla (1982), it is necessary to evaluate at least three dimensions: biological, social and psycho-affective - the latter two being rarely evaluated by health professionals. The biological dimension clearly appears in the reference to diseases, physiology and pathologies. The social dimension, in its strong reference to the social determinants of the population's health problems, is actually the consequences that the environment can have on an individual. The psycho-affective dimension is the strong appreciation of the symbolic component and the affective aspects involved in the act of healing and feeling healthy, in other words, self-care. It is with these three dimensions that the health professional must work in education, discarding the idea of the body as a machine, the dominance of the biological dimension over the others and neglecting the psychological, social and environmental aspects of the disease. Understanding the health-disease process as a result of living and working conditions means looking for ways to understand how it rebels in the collective. Not only health professionals but also citizens and public institutions must be involved in this effort.

In fact, health is a concept to be understood, so health is not taught, it is discussed: the relationship between health and living conditions, the right of the entire population to live in adequate conditions and so on (COLLARES et al, 1989). According to Alves (2005), p. 82, *"... to educate, to develop the art of thinking..."*.

It is well known that many diseases are in the community's own domain, meaning that the community itself could interfere with the problem, provided it is guided and prepared to do so. The population itself can then help with health programs at the level of prevention and, sometimes, cure. This gets to the root of the problem: keeping people away from illness and enabling them to achieve health and, consequently, improve their quality of life (CADERNOS DE EDUCAÇÂ POPULAR 7, 1984). This reasoning could be applied to improve the oral health of many communities.

However, according to Mendes (1992), dental teaching still reproduces retrograde elements such as: the structuring of the course plan in micro-disciplines and dental specialties, the general orientation of the curriculum still directed towards the lesion of the disease, with an emphasis on curative and rehabilitative, educational planning exclusively carried out by teachers, the nature of teaching staff and research.

According to Amaral (1991), although the number of colleges has increased over the last two decades in the country, the quality of oral health has not improved. This is because the current teaching model is incapable of providing health care for a large part of the population. University education is very deficient in relation to subjects that deal with social and preventive aspects, often leading to a lack of interest on the part of future professionals. In this sense, adds Alonso (1990), the university must take on the role of reflecting on what it is producing and reproducing as a transforming element with a commitment to society.

According to Valença (1992), educational work based on participation must go beyond the academic training that dental surgeons bring from university, moving towards a more comprehensive understanding of reality. It is from this perspective that dentists should be trained: to become health-promoting agents.

According to Barata et al. (1997), Cangussu et al. (2001) and Saliba (2003) et al., health is promoted by ensuring that citizens have decent living conditions through education, the adoption of healthy lifestyles, the development of individual skills and abilities, the production of a healthy environment, the implementation of public policies aimed at quality of life and health services. The vast majority of the causes of illness and disability could be avoided through preventive actions, provided that these activities were valued and linked to the population. As for curative and assistance measures, aimed at recovering individual health, they should only complement comprehensive health care (ROUQUAYROL, 1993). It is in this scenario that health education can play an important role: promoting the process of awareness of the right to health and providing tools for individual and collective intervention in the conditioning factors of the health/disease process (BRASIL, 1998).

For Aquilante et al. (2003), Batista (2005), Brasil (1998), Ferreira et al. (2004), Garcia et al. (2003) and Saliba et al. (2003), education and health are closely related and, in particular, health education is the result of the confluence of these two phenomena. In fact, educational action cannot be separated from health action, because the former is implicit in the latter and has objectives and goals based on the health situation of a population, which in turn reflects their living conditions. Education and health should be mutually reinforcing (AQUILANTE et al., 2003; BATISTA, 2005; FERREIRA et al., 2004; GARCIA et al., 2003; WHO, 1998; SALIBA et al., 2003), since limitations in either are obstacles to the full realization of human potential (MINAYO, 2000).

However, the dental surgeon's educational practice, understood as one of the components of basic health actions, is to provide people with the opportunity to develop a critical conscience, enabling them to take charge of solving their health problems (ROCHA 1989 and VALENÇA, 1992): not by telling them what is important to them, but by facilitating the conditions for them to see the importance of things (AQUILANTE et al., 2003; BATISTA, 2005; FERREIRA et al., 2004; GARCIA et al., 2003; WHO, 1998; PILON, 1986; SALIBA et al., 2003; VENTURA, 1989).

Aquilante et al. (2003), Batista (2005), Ferreira et al. (2004), Garcia et al. (2003), Saliba et al. (2003) and Valença (1992), state that traditional health education, within a hygienist conception, becomes a strange, alienating language, as it tends to be directed towards this or that behavior, forgetting its meaning in the context of the subject's life. When it stops being a process of persuasion or the transfer of education, it becomes a process of empowering individuals and groups to transform reality. In this process, the real participation of those involved must be sought, including the population and health professionals (AQUILANTE et al., 2003; BATISTA, 2005; FERREIRA et al., 2004; GARCIA et al., 2003; WHO, 1998; ROCHA, 1989; SALIBA et al., 2003).

Health education is a fundamental strategy in the process of forming behaviors that promote and maintain health, since through it it is possible to transform attitudes and behaviors, forming habits in the population to benefit their own health. It should be stressed that oral health education must be effective in improving individuals' knowledge and, consequently, changing their behavior (AQUILANTE et al., 2003; BATISTA, 2005; FERREIRA et al., 2004; GARCIA et al., 2003; WHO, 1998; SALIBA et al., 2003).

Thus, health education is one of the pillars of health promotion, which aims to empower and give people the opportunity to exercise control and improve their health. Health education actions should be associated with public health policies, clinical actions and community development (PORTILLO, 2000).

In communities, the school is an important center for teaching, learning, coexistence and growth, and fundamental vital values are shared there. It is therefore an ideal place to implement far-reaching and impactful health promotion programs, as it has a great influence on children during the most important formative stages of their lives (WHO, 1998).

Although school represents a very small sector in terms of time, given that the average student spends five hours a day in school, in the modern world its responsibilities are increasingly expanding, i.e. new responsibilities are being passed on to the school. It is often the school and the teachers who make immunization possible, the early detection of diseases in children, the improvement of sanitation and the organization of a whole range of primary health care activities (WHO, 1998). Health issues are becoming increasingly necessary to discuss in the school environment.

In health education, the teacher's most important role is that of a motivator who introduces the problems at hand, searches for information and support materials, problematizes and facilitates discussions by formulating strategies for school work (BRASIL, 1998). It is therefore important for teachers to be prepared to discuss health, hygiene and food issues in a critical and contextualized way, linking health to living conditions and citizens' rights (COLLARES, 1989). Developing a critical sense and shaping tomorrow's citizen is the task of education (COLLARES, 1989). Health education is a viable tool that should be used by educators to promote quality of life in Brazilian society (LOUREIRO, 1996). Rossetti (1999), p.105, also highlights the fact that professionals in the social field have greater methodological mastery and ideological commitment in the search for school-community-health service links, which favors health promotion in the school environment:

"*When* the *teacher teaches, he does so naturally, professionally; the teacher's knowledge is true, and he is believed, he is an example and a reference point. In contrast, the dentist is a stranger, with no pedagogical preparation for each child and their intellectual level, which is often feared and viewed with suspicion."*

Brito Bastos (1979) showed how knowledge can be integrated: through direct action by teachers on students, direct action on parents and indirect action by the students themselves on their parents, which would allow knowledge to spread, benefiting the whole community.

The action of a health program in the school environment brings a holistic view of the human being, considering people and especially children within their family, community and social environment (WHO, 1998).

Health promotion at school offers a valuable opportunity to distribute health knowledge, create hygienic habits and promote healthy lifestyles. Failing to take advantage of it is tantamount to running the risk of more and more children adopting unhealthy behaviors in the future, such as smoking, consuming alcohol and drugs and practicing dangerous sexual behavior at an early age or without adequate protection (WHO, 1998).

Each school is a particular combination of physical, cultural, emotional and social elements that give it a special character and define the teaching-learning process, determining the quality of the education that is delivered (WHO, 1998).

However, the school environment cannot be alienated from this important issue: health. An alienated school is one that forgets about the child's world outside the school environment and is concerned, according to Rossetti (1999), p.19, *"only with the child learning mathematics, history or biology and not with learning content about their own health".* Although the position can be defended that schools should not take on excessive responsibilities, since they are a manifestation of more complex social issues, they affect children and adolescents in particular, and it is precisely in the school environment, through education and other complementary interventions, that it has become possible to prevent many risk behaviors (WHO, 1998 and ROSSETTI, 1999). In this way, schools can carry out educational activities in relation to other health problems that arise in the regions, such as nutritional deficiencies, dental problems, vaccine-preventable diseases and malaria, among others (WHO, 1998).

According to Cabral (1998), people need to be highly motivated to acquire new health and citizenship habits and the professional must be technically and emotionally prepared for this work, since motivation involves a series of issues: empathy, responsibility, technical and scientific knowledge, availability, pleasure and involvement with political and social causes.

In order to help individuals with their needs to maintain and seek health, it is essential to get to know them through their reality, their way of life, beliefs, values, desires, how they organize themselves in the community, how they solve their individual and collective problems, how they get sick, how they treat their illness, how they use their bodies, their concept of quality of life and their expectation of having illness or health (PETTRY, 1997).

When they start school, children bring with them an appreciation of health-related behaviors from their families, other groups with more direct relationships or the media. However, in the pre-school years, children acquire the foundations of their behavior and knowledge, their sense of responsibility and the ability to observe, think and act, as well as adopt hygienic habits that will often last a lifetime, they also discover the potential of their bodies and develop skills and abilities to take care of their health and collaborate in the care of their family and community (WHO, 1998).

During childhood, a decisive time in the construction of behaviors, the school takes on a prominent role due to its potential for developing systematic and continuous work. It therefore needs to explicitly assume responsibility for health education, since the shaping of attitudes will be strongly associated with the values that the teacher and the entire school community will inevitably pass on to the pupils during everyday life (BRASIL, 1998). After all, according to Piotto (1998), there are many people involved and interested in early childhood education: children, families, educators, researchers, government and society - each with their own understanding of the quality of education.

Therefore, the development of educational and preventive programs that encourage and control behavior change is extremely important (HILL *et al.*, 2001; MWANGOSI, 2002; PETTRY et al., 1997).

In order to be effective and promote the incorporation of healthy habits, according to Harrison (2003), programs must be sensitive to the social and cultural differences of the target population and, consequently, take into account aspects such as: the use of specific language, continuity of information and clear and objective educational methods.

Educational methods should be used to make learning more enjoyable, attractive, meaningful and stimulating, especially when working with children (HARRISON, 2003; MASTRANTONIO, 2002; SANTOS, 2002).

Motivation and health education are therefore extremely important in promoting the oral health of the population. To this end, they should be worked on as early as possible and school age is a good time to work on motivation, because as well as manual skills, children have already developed a sense of cause/effect relationships, helping them to recognize the importance of prevention (SALIBA et al., 2003).

The success of preventive work is directly related to multiplier agents, i.e. individuals who learn, apprehend and pass on knowledge. Studies have shown that schoolchildren can be health multipliers, since they are able to apply the experiences they have had at school to their practical lives and pass them on to their families (GARCIA, 2003). It is based on these ideas that this work aims to act.

2.2 Health promoting school

Although educating for health is the responsibility of many other bodies, especially the health services themselves, the school is still the institution that can become a genuine space for promoting health (AQUILANTE et al., 2003; BATISTA, 2005; FERREIRA et al., 2004; FREIRE, 1995; GARCIA et al., 2003; SALIBA et al., 2003). After all, healthy children learn better, in addition to the fact that health problems compromise school attendance and, consequently, school performance (NOVA EDIÇÂO PEDAGÒGICA PARA A ESCOLA MODERNA, 1989 and WHO, 1998). It is true that places with more educated people have better health and quality of life, both for adults and children (BRASIL, 1998; WHO, 1998).

Normally, schools approach the issue of health from a biological point of view, in other words, the predominant themes of health lessons are diseases. And despite receiving information about specific ways of protecting themselves against each disease they study, students find it difficult to apply this information to concrete situations in their daily lives. In the same way, when the emphasis is on the disease and valuing individual behaviors that can prevent it, there is little room to build the student's conviction that the living conditions that favor the onset of diseases can also be modified (BRASIL, 1998). Therefore, it is clear that the aforementioned educational methodology has not proved sufficient for students to develop and adopt the behaviors and attitudes necessary health promotion, so how should the school redirect its actions in this area?

In fact, according to Figueiredo (2002), health care would be a complement to educational action, and the planning and implementation of these actions could take place in parallel with the planning of educational actions, since the school is an excellent communication channel for carrying out activities and transmitting health messages and serves as a distribution point for health services, in other words, establishing a link between learning at school and behavior outside of it (WHO, 1998). In fact, few settings offer, like schools, the possibility of generating integral commitments around the health initiative (AQUILANTE et al., 2003; FIGUEIREDO, 2002). After all, the development of verbal and written communication, for example, a priority in elementary school, is an essential element in the fight for health: when deciphering messages from educational programs and the media in general, when reading a prescription or a medicine leaflet, when understanding health as a right, or when seeking to improve the quality of service provision (BRASIL, 1998; NÓVOA, 1997). This is health education.

Despite what has been said above, why is it that the subject of health is still so little worked on in schools? After all, the topic of health has been highlighted as a cross-curricular theme that should be worked on, as far as possible, by all curricular subjects, and does not require specialized training. Specialized training is not necessary because the subject is present in people's daily lives and is easily accessible (BRASIL, 1998). After all, there aren't textbooks and teaching materials for all subjects, so what's the problem with tackling the issue of health at school?

So the idea is quite clear: when a school wants to commit itself to the health education of its students, in addition to functioning as a space that offers strong references for the practice and development of healthy lifestyles, it also includes the approach to the theme of health in the different curricular components, i.e. students will not only learn Portuguese, Mathematics, Science and other subjects, they will actually be able to use their knowledge to formulate real issues and problems. Therefore, a school should not just restrict itself to imposing content, in fact its main function is to educate its students for life (BOLIVAR, 1997 and BRASIL, 1998 and FREIRE, 1989).

Schools that have a safe and comfortable building, adequate drinking water and sanitary facilities and a positive psychological atmosphere for learning, that promote healthy human development and constructive and harmonious human relationships, and that promote positive health skills and attitudes, are therefore considered to be health-promoting schools (AQUILANTE et al., 2003 and WHO, 1998).

A significant part of the role of these schools is to impart knowledge and skills that promote self-care and help prevent risky behavior. Their activities are aimed at training young people with a critical spirit, capable of reflecting on the values, social situation and ways of life that are conducive to health and human development (WHO, 1998).

Health-promoting schools are therefore the ideal environment to raise children's awareness of the importance of physical and mental health and to pass on fundamental values, including the teaching of harmonious coexistence and respect for values and ways of relating to health that are different from their own (AQUILANTE et al., 2003 and WHO, 1998).

As children's or adolescents' health problems increase in frequency and severity, and their absence from school also increases, there is a growing need for the school to contribute to prevention programs, since the home on its own may not be capable of fulfilling this mission, given the complexity of the problems they face. Although the role of the family in the child's upbringing must be considered irreparable, the school can play a significant role in remedying some of the shortcomings of this stage of life. It is a question of seeking alliances between schools, families and the public sector in order to put common strategies into practice (BUSS, 1999; MARANHAO, 2000 and WHO, 1998).

Health-promoting schools should instill a sense of social responsibility in children and young people, developing their ability to resolve conflicts through dialogue and negotiation as a preventative factor against violence and an instrument for harmonious coexistence. Children and young people want to feel useful and are willing to work in the community, in hospitals, with the elderly or with younger children. These activities stimulate their social and community spirit and commitment, while allowing them to make constructive use of their free time, and are more effective the more they are integrated into the school learning process (WHO, 1998).

Therefore, it is not up to the teacher to dictate rules of behavior or to act as a role model. It's up to them to develop children's critical sense, so that they can identify problems and seek original and creative answers to them.

However, it is not possible to separate the attitudes and procedures of care aimed at education from the attitudes and procedures aimed at health promotion, just as it is not possible to separate the biological from the cultural and affective (MARANHAO, 2000).

2.3 ***Psychomotricity and Playfulness***

Psychomotricity is understood as the science whose object of study is man through his body in movement and in relation to his internal and external world, as well as his possibilities for perceiving, acting, acting with others, with objects and with himself (ALMEIDA, 1994; BERGE, 1968; CAVALLARI et al, 1994; CHÂTEAU, 1987; FAZIO, 2000; HAYDT, 1998; KHISHIMOTO, 1994; MACHADO, 1994; OAKLANDER, 1980; SILVA, 1997; MALUF, 2003; RODRIGUES, 1992; WEISS, 1997). There is a close parallel between the development of motor functions and the development of psychic functions. In other words, the more numerous and richer the situations experienced by the child, the greater the number of schemes they acquire. In this way, psychomotricity, as a science of education, seeks to educate movement at the same time as developing the functions of intelligence (MALUF, 2003).

The development of body awareness, reflection and creativity, as well as full affective, cognitive and motor development, are some of the objectives of psychomotricity which, if achieved, will lead to healthy and happy adults. Therefore, providing psychomotor work will help structure the child's personality, as they can better express their desires, work out their fantasies, develop their needs and work through their difficulties. As has already been said, psychomotricity is a science which, because it has man as the object of its study, encompasses several other areas: education, pedagogy and health, which is the issue we intend to focus on in this work. Psychomotricity takes into account the communicative aspect of the human being, the body and gestures, with the aim of making the individual: a being of communication, creation and operative thought (ALMEIDA, 1994; BERGE, 1968; CAVALLARI et al.,1994CHÂTEAU, 1987; FAZIO, 2000; HAYDT, 1998; KHISHIMOTO, 1994; MACHADO, 1994; MALUF, 2003; OAKLANDER, 1980; RODRIGUES, 1992; SILVA, 1997; WEISS, 1997).

Relational concepts permeate the individual's relationships of desire, frustration, action and interaction with the environment, with space, with objects and with themselves - characteristics and experiences that are easily experienced and interpreted by children during play activities (ALMEIDA, 1994; BERGE, 1968; CAVALLARI et al.,1994CHÂTEAU, 1987; FAZIO, 2000; HAYDT, 1998; KHISHIMOTO, 1994; MACHADO, 1994; MALUF,2003; OAKLANDER,1980; RODRIGUES, 1992; SILVA, 1997; WEISS,1997).

For a long time, researchers, educators, psychologists and other scholars have been highlighting the importance of games and play for children's education. Major contributions have already been made and the conclusion has been reached that through play children make new discoveries and challenges and that their development is enhanced (VIEIRA et al., 2005 and VYGOTSKY, 1988).

Man, par excellence, has always shown a playful tendency to carry out his tasks, using play in education, associating the idea of study with pleasure. The importance of sensory education has therefore determined the use of "didactic play" by teachers in the most diverse areas, such as philosophy, mathematics, language study and other subjects. However, from a very early age, a child's essential activity is to play, and in this way they are able to express themselves and communicate, becoming a social being. In fact, play is a device that children use to interact and thus establish new roles in their relationship with the world (BROUGÉRE, 1998).

Play for the child is not the same as play and fun for the adult, just leisure. Perhaps the main reason for the theft of play in childhood is that children are seen as miniature adults whose sole purpose is to prepare them for the future. However, the world of play, in essence, is not about systematic preparation for the future, but about living in the present, in the now. It is therefore necessary to understand the child as a producer of culture, giving them the time and space necessary for this production, ensuring they have the right to play, enabling a variety of experiences and contributing to their formation as a human being participating in the society in which they live. Although we talk about understanding the universe of children, what we actually see is the instrumentalization of childhood, which has been happening frequently, disrespecting the child's age group and pushing them further and further away from play and playfulness in their daily practice, with the school unfortunately being one of the contributors to this instrumentalization (MARCELLINO, 1996).

However, some parents are only concerned with formal learning and serious subjects, anxious about the child's cognitive and biological maturation. As a result, they end up preventing and disrespecting their children's play, expecting them to be disciplined, controlled and responsible (BERGE, 1968; BOLIVAR, 1997; NÓVOA, 1997).

Play is the child's work, a very serious thing, an activity through which they develop, discover social roles, their limits, try out new skills and form a new concept of themselves. By playing, they explore the world, make small rehearsals, gradually understand and assimilate its rules and patterns, and absorb this world in small, tolerable doses (BERGE, 1968; BROUGÉRE, 1998; CAVALLARI et al., 1994; CHÂTEAU, 1987; MALUF, 2003; HAYDT, 1998; KHISHIMOTO, 1994; OAKLANDER, 1980; RODRIGUES, 1992; SILVA, 1997; WEISS, 1997).

Games and play have changed a lot, but the pleasure of playing hasn't and, at the same time, play is both pleasurable and serious (BROUGÉRE, 1998; CHÂTEAU, 1987; KHISHIMOTO, 1994; WEISS, 1997). Play, like other traditions, is dynamic and is influenced by social evolution (MUNGUBA, 2002). Children need interesting and motivating options to participate in the world. In this respect, play has the potential to facilitate the fixation of visual and auditory perceptions because stimuli in these areas, with contrasts and geared towards children's interests, lead to assimilation (MUNGUBA, 2002 and PINTO, 1997).

Games are valuable not only because of the interest they universally arouse, or the joy that individuals experience in playing them, but also because they have an educational dimension in their context, because they have the great advantage of offering those who take part in them the opportunity for integral development, covering the physical, mental, emotional and social fields of the human being (BERGE, 1968; BROUGÉRE, 1998; CAVALLARI et al, 1994; CHÂTEAU, 1987; HAYDT, 1998; KHISHIMOTO, 1994; MALUF, 2003; OAKLANDER, 1980; RODRIGUES, 1992; SILVA, 1997; WEISS, 1997).

In addition, it is usually through games and play that children share their memories, constituting not only a type of informal education but also a kind of common cultural production. Children construct their social worlds, in other words, they construct their surroundings and the wider society in which they live (BROUGÉRE, 1998; PINTO, 1997).

Imagination is a new psychological process for the child; it represents a specifically human form of conscious activity, and play promotes this imaginary situation, and teaches the child to direct their behavior not only by the immediate perception of objects or the situation, but by the meaning of the situation (REGO, 2001).

In playful activity, what matters is not just the product of the activity, what results from it, but the action itself, the moment lived. It allows those who experience it to have moments of encounter with themselves and with others, moments of fantasy and reality, of meaning and perception, moments of self-knowledge and knowledge of others, of taking care of oneself and looking at others, moments of life (POLETTO, 2005).

Recent studies have also shown that play activities are indispensable tools in child development, because for children there is no activity more complete than playing. Through play, the child is introduced into the sociocultural environment of the adult, constituting a way of assimilating and recreating reality (SANTOS, 1999).

Children need to be involved in the act of playing in order to be able to organize their ideas and thus externalize their deepest feelings, which will allow them to always be placed in challenges and situations that will help them to improve the very construction of their learning. In this sense, playing is also a great channel for learning, if not the only channel for real cognitive processes (MACHADO, 1994; MEDEIROS JÛNIOR et al., 2005). One extraordinary ability that we use all the time, but are not aware of, is the ability to construct virtual realities in our heads.

Therefore, playfulness helps considerably in the child's knowledge and cognitive development, by seeking interaction between the adult world and the child's world (MACHADO, 1994; NEIRA, 1990).

However, children interact through play, since through their minds they create and recreate passages from their lives, making connections with events and facts that narrate their daily lives (MARANHAO, 2003 and MEDEIROS JÛNIOR et al., 2005).

Playful activity plays an important educational role in children's development, as they develop, get to know and construct the world, based on social exchanges, the different life stories of children, parents and teachers, which is strengthened by family interaction, incorporated into the school. It's easier to work with students in a child and adolescent health promotion program when the school-student-family triad is aligned in its purposes and expectations (ROCHA, 2000 and SANTOS, 1999).

Given this context, it is understood that learning through recreation is extremely habitual for children, as this action is part of their competence, enabling them to enter their world with the aim of collecting important information that will contribute to designing and developing activities inherent to their roles and aimed at their underlying areas of need (FAZIO, 2000 and FORTUNA, 2001).

With this, children, who are the protagonists of their own learning, can incorporate a more active dynamic, with a greater tendency to learn meaningfully (BRASIL, 1998; COSTA et al., 1997). It could also be said that games are children's favorite activities. All they have to do is get two or three of them together and there they are kicking a ball, trying to see who can jump or balance better or making guesses. If there are no rules, they create them, if there are no suitable materials, they improvise them, and that's how they learn: by playing.

This is easily perceived by simply observing the pleasure that a small group is getting out of a game (BERGE, 1968; BROUGÉRE, 1998; CAVALLARI et al., 1994; CHÂTEAU, 1987; HAYDT, 1998; KHISHIMOTO, 1994; MALUF, 2003; OAKLANDER, 1980; RODRIGUES, 1992; SILVA, 1997; WEISS,1997).

According to Duarte Júnior, p. 67, 1995, *"education is certainly a profoundly aesthetic and creative activity in itself. It has the meaning of a game, of a toy, in which we involve ourselves pleasurably in search of harmony".* The aim here is to describe a dynamic way of working in health: ludo-education.

3. Justification

Health education programs lead individuals to have correct information and participatory attitudes in educational actions, thus improving their health conditions, quality of life and consequently their citizenship (BARROS, 1996). However, there is an urgent need to complement education with health teaching, in other words, to strengthen and transform schools (WHO, 1998). To do this, it is not necessary to have a teacher or other specialist professional, but rather to focus on the value of pedagogical work whose main focus is on health and not on illness. To this end, it is necessary to raise awareness and encourage the participation of the population so that oral health improves significantly. In this sense, it is necessary to work on motivating people to change their habits, raise awareness of their rights and demand that they do so (BATISTA, 2005).

This work aims to become a health-promoting agent capable of changing beliefs, attitudes and erroneous behavior in relation to health practiced by a large part of the population. This study is justified by the great need to introduce in Brazil, especially in poor communities, the awareness of the population of the importance of preventive procedures in relation to health, not only physical, but also mental. By introducing strategies related to general and oral health, the aim was to teach the target group about the possibility of avoiding illness by changing inappropriate habits, making them carriers of health knowledge.

We are fighting for health, for quality of life, after all, according to Alves (2005), p.15, *"Life is not justified by utility. It is justified by pleasure and joy.*

Just as a patient needs individual treatment, a community also needs it, organizing itself for its own health: *"A health plan is not just an action that is set in motion, it must have continuity"* (ROSSETTI, p.124, 1999).

4. Objectives

4.1 General objective

The aim of this study is to develop, through a theoretical and scientific basis, a more comprehensive model for analyzing the health-disease phenomenon, which prioritizes the understanding of health as a collective value, of social determination, in other words, moving from a model of care, centered on disease and based on providing care to those who seek it, to a model of comprehensive health care.

4.2 Specific objectives

- Offering future professionals contact with the reality in which they will be working, as well as strengthening university-community ties;
- Encouraging interdisciplinary work, focusing on the importance of future professionals learning to work as part of a team;
- To educate about the various aspects of a healthy life and to help clarify misconceptions or superstitions that conspire against health;
- Making children carriers of knowledge;
- Raising awareness of the importance of prevention education;
- To understand the practice of childcare workers in an educational context, from the point of view of health, as well as working with them, where necessary, to re-evaluate their concepts and raise awareness of the responsibility they have for their children in terms of practicing healthy habits;
- To verify the effect of a self-instruction method on oral and general health knowledge applied to schoolchildren of different socioeconomic levels;
- Propose simple, low-cost educational and motivational strategies;
- Ensuring a healthy environment for students, as well as creating school hours of pleasure, fun and learning;
- Monitoring and helping to improve students' nutritional status;
- Providing schoolchildren with a better level of knowledge about general and oral health, combining education with pleasure;
- Aiming for a better relationship between schoolchildren and health professionals;

- Demystifying inadequate beliefs, attitudes and behaviors in relation to health;
- Converting those being treated from a passive position to an active attitude towards their own health;
- Promoting physical and mental health for all those involved, teachers, staff and students.

5. Methodology

5.1 Line of research

The aim is to develop an educational model aimed at teaching people about the health-disease process and, above all, its determinants and preventive resources. The aim is to propose a methodology that reaches everyone equally, without excluding race, gender, physical or mental disability, economic situation or geographical location, seeking to reduce the inequalities of access that are often observed. One of the most effective ways of achieving this is through health promotion in schools: health education.

5.2 Work team

The success of a job is directly related to the capacity and competence of a team. According to Alves (2005), p. 79, *"Competence has to do with the ability to solve real problems, situations as they appear in life"*. The aim here is to encourage the involvement and participation of the entire work team in the program, where they will act to help integrate health and education, offering full attention to the child. An interdisciplinary team is needed: dentistry, psychology, social work and pedagogy. The members should be chosen with the aim of highlighting the importance of interdisciplinarity, an issue that is still little discussed and, above all, practiced in academic circles - after all, oral health is not just a problem to be assessed by a dentist. It will therefore be up to the members to develop and carry out the dynamic activities in the schools.

5.3 Target population

This work will be carried out in a school environment. It should be applied to duly enrolled school-age children, including teachers, preparing them for the development of the pedagogical project that requires the inclusion of content related to health promotion and improving the quality of services provided to children. Although it takes place in the school, the intention is to turn those being assisted into carriers of information and, consequently, to take this information back to their families, their neighborhoods, their communities and so on, in other words, making health a collective issue.

In fact, the aim is to train those being assisted to become community health agents. According to the Ministry of Health (1999), a community health worker is a worker who is part of the health team in the community where they live. They are trained to welcome families and advise them on caring for their own health and that of the community in which they live. Undoubtedly, this worker has special characteristics, since he works in the same community where he lives, making the relationship between work and social life stronger.

Therefore, it can be summarized that by applying this methodology, the following will be achieved:

- **School-age children** of both sexes, from four to six years old, with one group made up of children from a public school and the other from a private school. Children at this age are more suited to motivational work because, in addition to manual skills, they have already developed a sense of cause/effect relationships, helping them to recognize the importance of prevention (RODRIGUES, 1992);

- **Children's educators**, re-evaluating their concepts of health and making them aware of the responsibility they have towards children in terms of practicing healthy habits. After all, the figure of the teacher has a great influence on the behavior of the students, due to their daily contact over a long period of time (SANTOS, 2002);

- The **families of those being assisted**, which will be an evaluation of the effectiveness of the method, testing the effectiveness of the information provided by the children;

- **Volunteer** members of the project, who will be trained here to work in a multidisciplinary team.

5.4 Workplace

Schools are the ideal place to develop educational and preventive programs, as they allow all children to have access to them, including those who, for whatever reason, do not have access to private professional care (WHO, 1998). It is also in the school environment that children are introduced to a collective environment. As a result, the school served will be differentiated by its characteristics[1] and will be called a "Health Promoting School".

5.5 Action strategies

This work will be developed through dynamic activities that should be developed in one year and didactically divided into two semesters.

The first semester will be aimed at introducing the children to each other and forming an intimate bond with them. This proposal aims to show them that the dental surgeon is not just a professional who cares for and treats oral health, but also plays, talks and, above all, can be a friend and companion. The aim of the project is not only to teach, but also to ensure that information is learned and passed on, offering care and pleasure to those being treated.

A number of goals will be developed for the first semester, divided into eight stages:

- Step 1: **Presentation (In search of "Health Warriors")**;
- Stage 2: **Good manners**;
- Stage 3: **My house**;
- Stage 4: **My family**;
- Stage 5: **Habits and notions of hygiene**;
- Stage 6: **Sense organs**;
- Stage 7: **Food and Nutrition**;
- Step 8: **Preventing domestic accidents**.

All these stages should be worked through in a playful way. Paying attention to the individuality of each child, checking for attention, interest, learning and, above all, apprehension. This way, the child will not only be able to use the knowledge for themselves, but also pass it on to their family, neighborhood, community and so on, which will achieve the goal of making them multipliers of knowledge.

After this first phase, the second semester will focus more on the issue of oral health. This methodology was chosen in the belief that this would demystify the fear that children usually have of health professionals, which makes them known to dentists and dental students as difficult to treat. In the general population, almost 7% said they were very afraid of the service, while another 13% said they felt some fear. In Brazil, a prevalence of 15% of dental anxiety sufferers was found. Other studies have also found an association between fear and poor oral health (KANEGANE et al., 2003).

It's worth noting that the first semester will serve as a bridge between the team members and those they serve - who until then would have seen them only as fellow health workers.

Before starting the second semester's activities, we recommend setting up a exhibition of photographs, drawings, diagrams and a review of everything that was worked on in the first phase of the project. This display would be placed in a place that is easily accessible to everyone in the school. The children would then see themselves in the photos, admire their work and become more motivated for the second stage.

As in the first semester, the second semester will also follow these targets:

- Step 9ª: **Dentists and doctors are our friends**;
- Stage 10: **Teeth and their functions**;
- Stage 1: **Caries and Periodontal Disease**;

- Step 12: **Toothbrush**;
- 13th step: **Toothpaste and dental floss**;
- Step 14: **Brushing my teeth**;
- Stage 15: **The Plate Developer and The Flûor**;
- Stage 16: **Closing**.

In order to ensure communication and adherence to the process by parents and/or guardians, each child should have a notebook, **Caderno da Saù (Health Notebook**), where pamphlets will be posted with all the information covered, with the aim of reinforcing at home the topics covered in the school environment.

This is the context in which this project intends to operate, aiming to work on health education in a playful way, considering this activity to be a fertile cradle for the child's intellectual activities, and indispensable to educational practice (ALMEIDA, 1994; CAVALLARI, 1994; CHÂTEAU, 1987; KHISHIMOTO, 1994; MACHADO, 1994; OAKLANDER, 1980; RIZZI et al, 1998; RODRIGUES, 1992; WEISS, 1997). For this reason, it will be the members' concern to use vocabulary and techniques that are accessible to both the age group and the socio-economic conditions of the group served.

5.6 Period/Schedule

This work will last one year, and the practical and theoretical activities will be carried out in accordance with the school timetable of both the students and the members of the study.

First semester

Table 1: Distribution of dynamic activities for the first semester.

Activities	*March April*	*May*	*June*
Step 1ª: **Presentation**	X		
Step 2ª: **Good manners**	X		
3ª stage: **My house**	X		
4ª step: **My family**	X		
Stage 5: **Habits and notions of hygiene**		X	
Stage 6: **Sense organs**		X	
Stage 7: **Food and Nutrition**			X

Step 8: **Preventing domestic accidents**				X

Second semester

Table 2: Distribution of dynamic activities for the second semester.

Activities	***August***	***Sep.***	***Oct.***	***Nov.***
Step 9: **Dentists and doctors are our friends**	X			
Step 10ª: **Teeth and their functions**	X			
Step 11ª: **Caries and Periodontal Disease**		X		
12ª step: **Toothbrush**		X		
Step 13: **Toothpaste and dental floss**			X	
Step 14: **Brushing my teeth**			X	
Stage 15: **The Plate Developer and The Flûor**				X
Stage 16: **Closing**				X

6. Result indicators

Some questions arise here: how do you evaluate a project developed and based on a qualitative methodology? What procedures should be adopted to evaluate the art of thinking, love or even happiness? After all, it would be impossible to conclude that someone is 23.46% happy, 74.39% in love and that only 2.15% of the group surveyed is unhappy - unfortunately, there are still no multiple choice evaluations for happiness. The indices that have been used so far are exclusively for measuring illness, disregarding the social and psycho-affective issues of the group studied. After all, education in itself is an indicator of health: the more people study, the better they are able to fight disease and preserve their health (MEDRONHO, 2002 and ROUQUAYROL, 1993). It would be useful here to construct indices that assess what has actually been learned. According to Alves (2005), p.72-74:

ªWhat has really been learned is what has survived the purifying action of forgetting. What has been learned is what remains after oblivion has done its work... Only the knowledge that makes sense will remain... Memory keeps what has given pleasure... Memory is intelligent and forgets what doesn't make sense".

As quoted by the WHO (1998), p.11:

"In fact, the teaching-learning process should be constantly evaluated with the participation not only of the project's executors, but also of teachers, parents, students and, if possible, community representatives."

Therefore, the best resource here would be **common sense**, with the members being able to assess the students according to a number of domains: **affective**, **psychomotor** and **cognitive**. In the first, affective assessment, the focus should be on how much the schoolchild appreciates the program, whether they participate actively and with motivation in the programmed events and whether they value their oral health. In terms of psychomotor skills, the aim is to ensure adequate mechanical control of plaque. In terms of cognition, the aim is to assess understanding of the causes and consequences of oral problems and the means of preventing and controlling them. For this last assessment, four questionnaires will have to be developed that address the information passed on to the children: for the children, for the school staff, another for the families and a final one for the project members. Through these questionnaires, not only will the learning of those assisted be assessed, but also their ability to pass on information.

6.1 *Child assessment*

The same children's questionnaire will be administered three times:

- At the beginning of the project (Stage 1), questions will be asked about all the stages. This will make it possible to assess the children's current health knowledge;

- At the end of the first semester, the same questionnaire should be applied, i.e. with all the questions relating to the topics that have been and will be worked on, analyzing possible progress in assimilation in relation to the topics worked on;

- At the end of the second semester, the same questionnaire is repeated when all the topics have been covered, assessing the final level of knowledge acquired by those involved.

6.2 *Family assessment*

The family assessment will be carried out using a questionnaire, administered twice:

- At the beginning of the project, to assess current knowledge of the topics to be covered;

- At the end of the project, the capacity of the children will be evaluated as carriers of knowledge, comparing the results obtained from the first application of the questionnaire with the last.

6.3 *Evaluation of school staff*

The evaluation of the school staff will be very similar to that of the family. The questionnaire will be administered twice:

- At the beginning of the project, it served as a resource to assess the current knowledge of the school team in relation to the topics to be addressed, as well as directing the team in the orientation and demystification of health issues;

- At the end of the work, by evaluating whether or not they were satisfied, the children's capacity as carriers of knowledge will be assessed, comparing the results obtained from the first application of the questionnaire with the last.

6.4 *Evaluation of project members*

The evaluation of the project members will begin with the selection of the team, which will have to undergo a theoretical-scientific evaluation, a curriculum evaluation and an interview. In addition, it will be up to those selected to provide a weekly report on each stage worked in the school environment, and they will also be responsible for further evaluation and discussion of the reports among the team formed, in order to work out possible problems to be faced - after all, solutions can emerge from conversations and discussions. The aim is to ensure greater efficiency in the execution of this work.

7. Description and discussion of ideas

The population directly affected will be schoolchildren, who will be divided into groups corresponding to the number of classrooms, each of which will be visited weekly. The project can be carried out in any school, public or private, so there will be no social, economic or cultural exclusion.

Health education will be introduced and evaluated during the project, which will have two main phases. The first will be aimed at introducing the children to each other and creating an intimate bond with them. The second will focus more on oral health issues. Both phases will be divided into stages, which will be described and discussed later.

All these stages will be worked through in a playful way. This methodology is chosen because there is a close parallel between the development of motor functions and the development of psychic functions. In other words, the more numerous and richer the situations experienced by the child, the greater the number of schemes they acquire. In this way, psychomotricity, as a science of education, seeks to educate movement at the same time as developing the functions of intelligence (ALMEIDA, 1994; CAVALLARI et al., 1994; CHÂTEAU , 1987; KHISHIMOTO, 1994; MACHADO, 1994; OAKLANDER, 1980; RIZZI et al, 1998; RODRIGUES, 1992; WEISS, 1997).

Thus, it is necessary to understand the child as a producer of culture, giving them the time and space necessary for this production, ensuring their right to play, enabling a variety of experiences and contributing to their formation as a human being participating in the society in which they live (ALMEIDA, 1994; CAVALLARI et al, 1994; CHÂTEAU , 1987; KHISHIMOTO, 1994; MACHADO, 1994; OAKLANDER, 1980; RIZZI et al, 1998; RODRIGUES, 1992; WEISS, 1997).

According to Machado, 1994, children need to be involved in the act of playing in order to be able to organize their ideas and thus externalize their deepest feelings, which allow them to always be placed in challenges and situations that make them improve the very construction of their learning. In this sense, play is also a great channel for learning, if not the only channel for real cognitive processes (ALMEIDA, 1994; CAVALLARI et al., 1994; CHÂTEAU , 1987; KHISHIMOTO, 1994; MACHADO, 1994; OAKLANDER, 1980; RIZZI et al, 1998; RODRIGUES, 1992; WEISS, 1997).

Given this context, it is understood that learning through recreation is extremely common in childhood, as this action is part of their competence, enabling them to enter their world with the aim of collecting important information that will contribute to designing and developing activities inherent to their roles and aimed at their underlying areas of need (FAZIO, 2000).

7.1 *Description of stages*

Each stage will be described here according to the objectives pursued. The dynamics for working on each proposal will also be described. As far as the materials needed to carry out the games and activities suggested are concerned, it will not be necessary to use sophisticated material, as the aim was to use only materials available in the school itself, or else low-cost materials, ensuring the accessibility of this work. Below is a description and discussion of each stage to be worked on.

First semester

1ª Stage: Presentation (in search of "health warriors")

I Objectives:

As already described, this work will develop its activities based on recreational techniques. Therefore, the project will be presented to the beneficiaries as a training ground aimed at forming "warriors" who will have to fight for their health and who will be trained to use "strategies" to preserve it.

It is recommended, however, that the team be introduced to each classroom in the school through the school staff, which would provide greater security for those involved, since the project members would be accompanied by figures known and respected by the school's students.

In front of the children, each member will be introduced and, as far as the educational method is concerned, they will be told the main reason why the team is looking for them: "THE WORLD IS LOOKING FOR WARRIORS". In fact, these "warriors" will be referred to as "Health Warriors". In order to guarantee and encourage adherence, each child will receive a card at the end of the project **(Annex I)**, for which they will have to undergo "training", where they will learn how to carry out and teach possible measures to improve their quality of life. In addition, at the end of the project, each classroom will be given a "certificate" **(Appendix II)** of completion of the project. In fact, the latter would "make" the bearer a "Health Warrior".

On the same day, each child should be given a notebook, which we will refer to here as the **"Health Notebook"**. A notice **(Annex III)** should be posted in this notebook, which should be taken to parents and/or guardians, explaining to them that their children will be part of an educational project, and requesting that this commitment form be signed in order to start the practical activities.

II Dynamic activities

Activity: Who am I?

The activity here is designed to stimulate children's logical thinking. They should work on self-esteem and awareness of the parts of their body and their usefulness, as well as the respect and care they need to take with their own bodies. Discuss with the children that when we are perfectly healthy we feel happy, rested, ready to play and study. Remind the children that they are developing and that the fact that they are constantly growing is also a sign of a well-functioning body. If an older child is uninterested in the activity, we recommend asking them to help and take part in the game - after all, older children need stimulation too.

- *Materials used:* sheets of manila paper, cardboard or newspaper; marker pens, crayons or colored pencils.
- *Instructions:* The children will be asked to draw the outline of their feet, hands and body. Encourage the children to add the missing details. Explore the concepts of "right/left". Stimulate the children's logical thinking by asking what each part of the body is for, for example, what are the hands and feet for? What are the teeth for? Afterwards, cut out the drawings and color them in to create a self-portrait with the outline of their own body.

III Discussion

The conclusion here is that the development of body awareness helps children to learn how the human body works and to appreciate the importance of a well-functioning body for life. This knowledge, however, is not an end in itself, but is the basis for achieving a healthy life guaranteed by a well-functioning body.

2ª Stage: Good manners

I Objectives

The aim of this stage is to make the children aware of the importance of having good manners, and that they exist to improve coexistence between people. The aim here will be to stimulate self-criticism and common sense, i.e. each child will evaluate their own attitudes and, if necessary, will be encouraged to change habits that are inconsistent with good socialization. This activity will also bring advantages to this study, as the children will be better prepared for the group dynamics.

II Dynamic activities

Activity: Theatrical fishing

As everyone knows, what you do on a fishing trip is catch fish. However, this will be a different activity, because each fish caught will carry a message, and it will be up to the children to interpret it.

- *Materials used:* large plastic bowl, sand, cardboard, felt-tip pens or colored pencils and a fishing rod.
- Instructions: Use the cardboard to make cut-outs of fish, which should be colored in with a hydro-graphic pen or colored pencils. These will contain proposals for topics such as: what to do when entering a room; how to speak; how to eat; what to do when seeing an elderly person getting on a bus and various other situations. Once the little fish are ready, they will be placed in a bowl filled with sand for the children to catch at random. Once the fish has been caught, the message it carries should be read out. At this point, it is up to the members of the project to interpret the situation brought up by the message. For example, if the topic drawn is "what should you do before entering the classroom?", two situations will be interpreted: in the first, the actors will enter shouting, pushing each other, without knocking on the door or asking permission from those in the room; in the other situation, they will do the opposite, i.e. they will arrive quietly, asking permission and greeting everyone in the room. The next step will be to stimulate the child's critical sense, asking them to evaluate each situation, discerning the correct attitude from the incorrect one.

III Discussion

This way of working with theatrical games in such a way as to always seek to overcome the challenges proposed can greatly help the individual to develop a sense of responsibility in relation to the environment in which they operate, be it at school, in the family, in the neighborhood, or in their group of friends.

Therefore, this activity aims to contribute to the development of a more critical thinking of the students in relation to the social reality in which they are inserted, by working various themes and discussions based on the theatrical games and scenes produced by the members of the project. Thus, through critical action, which considers and reflects on reality, we arrive at a theatrical educational activity committed to the intellectual evolution of man (NOVA EDIÇÂO PEDAGÒGICA PARA A ESCOLA MODERNA, 1989).

Thus, acting in theatrical games from an educational perspective can lead the individual to self-knowledge, to the development of skills that are essential for coexistence and growth in a group and to intervening in their community in a more conscious way. In this way, instead of simply reproducing the current social order in the fragmented formation of individuals, the school should pay greater attention to the more integral development of the learner, understanding them as a creative, dynamic and transforming being.

3ª Stage: My house

I Objectives:

The focus here will be on showing the children the importance of knowing the physical environment in which they live, as well as the importance of knowing the location of their house, showing that it has a number, that it is on a street and that it is in a neighborhood, which has a postal address code (C.E.P.) and is therefore in a city. In addition, this stage will help the members get an idea of the children's living conditions. The importance of the children carrying their identification with them, including the address and contact telephone number of their parents and/or guardians, should be discussed with them - taking advantage of the opportunity, the "card" that will be provided by the project will have all the data mentioned about the child (Annex I).

Afterwards, attention will be paid to the physical space in question, advising on the functions and care of the rooms in the house, for example, in the bedroom you sleep and keep your clothes; in the living room you usually watch TV and so on.

The children should be taught that a house should be clean and organized, and that everyone in the household should be responsible for preserving and cleaning it.

II Dynamic activities

Activity: My house is like this

In order to develop and reaffirm the concepts passed on to the children in relation to their homes, the activity will be carried out by making a "floor plan" of a house on cardboard. This will enable them to work out the physical space of a house, as well as working on their critical sense, since they will be actively participating in the game.

- *Materials used:* cardboard, illustrative cut-outs of household utensils (shower, sink, comb, stove, fridge, closet, bed, television, toys and others), pins (for attaching the cut-outs).
- Instructions: A schematic "floor plan" with a simplistic division of a house will be drawn on a piece of cardboard. Pictures of household utensils will be brought in and the children will be asked what they are, what they are for, where they should be in the house and how they should be kept. After explaining, it's up to the members to affix the picture to the correct place on the floor. For example, if the child has a picture of a shower. It will be up to the

project members to ask the child what the shower is for, whether it poses any risk of accidents and, of course, where the shower is.

this appliance must be installed.

Creating in children a basic sense of geographic location, organization and the active cooperation they can have with their own homes is what we believe we can achieve by applying this playful activity. After all, according to Haydt (1998), p. 6, *"it is through playing and games that children organize the world around them, assimilating experiences and information and, above all, incorporating activities and values"*.

4ª Stage: My family

I Objectives

According to Carvalho *et al.* (2003), the family is seen as a key element not only for the "survival" of individuals, but also for their protection and socialization, in addition to the transmission of cultural and economic capital and group property, as well as gender relations and solidarity between generations.

The influence of the family environment is often decisive for an individual's development, where parents and siblings continue to be the child's main socializing agents, especially in the early years.

The family and the school play important roles in the child's formation during the various stages of discovery in life, and it is up to them to accompany, protect, educate and encourage the child's early socialization. Consolidating this partnership is necessary, as the school-family interrelationship requires continuous coordination in order to strengthen and achieve goals aimed at building citizenship.

The aim here is to get to know not only the family (quantity), but also the family environment in which the children live (quality). Therefore, it should be made clear to those being assisted that, normally, a family is made up of a father, mother and siblings, but there are other types of family environments that have a stepfather or stepmother, or are headed by grandparents or uncles. In fact, the main focus will be on showing that family is not just a matter of kinship, but a condition of harmonious coexistence between the members of a household. In the end, however, it cannot be said that children who benefit from so-called "normal" family conditions have advantages over other family environments.

It is also important to question the profession of each family member and their importance. Another topic to be addressed will be the issue of violence: not just physical violence, but also verbal violence. Make the children aware of the importance of respect, cooperation and, above all, of spreading love and affection in the family environment.

II Dynamic activities

Activity: My family is important to me

The aim of this activity is to get to know each child's family better. This provides support for the members of the team to better direct subsequent activities, guaranteeing humanized, individualized and, consequently, more efficient work.

- *Materials used:* office paper, colored pencils, crepe paper and white glue.

- Instructions: it will be up to the members of the project to make cut-outs of dolls out of paper. These will be given to each child, where each member of the child's family will be represented by a doll. They will also be given crepe paper balls, colored pencils and glue. After the individual artistic work with each child, they will be asked what each doll represents in their family, what the relationship between them is and so on.

The purpose of this activity is to study and evaluate the families of the children in our care. After all, it is through the experiences that children have with the people in their family and with their friends at school that they learn the rules of social interaction, to respect the rights and wishes of others as much as their own.

Studying family relationships, observing your family, will awaken in the child the idea of social interdependence, making them feel that there is a need for cooperation and mutual help and that as a social member, each individual, just like them, has responsibilities.

5ª Stage: Habits and notions of hygiene

I Objectives:

As you know, proper hygiene habits are essential for avoiding many diseases and preserving health. It is therefore important to work on this valuable cause, approaching it in a logical way, following the child's daily chronology. It will be up to the members to interact with the children on an ongoing basis: the system of questions (What is it?, What is it for?, How do we do it?, Can we do it on our own?) and answers will help the students understand the importance of hygiene rules and the advantages they offer.

Several topics will be covered as follows: what we do to start the day well (stretching, washing our face, combing our hair, having a snack and brushing our teeth); what we use to bathe (water, soap, towel and sponge); how to clean our ears and nostrils (use of flexible sticks and handkerchiefs); clothing (cleanliness, what clothes to wear in hot and cold weather); during meals (washing hands, chewing food well, not talking while chewing and brushing teeth after meals); questioning sleep (hours, wearing pajamas, clean bedding). Addressing harmful habits (nail biting, sucking on fingers or nipples, putting objects in the mouth) - always questioning their harmful effects and stressing the importance of stopping them.

II Dynamic activities

Activity: surprise box (What is it? What is it for? How do I do it? Can I do it myself?)

The activity proposed here will not only reinforce concepts relating to good habits, but will also work with the children on how to carry them out correctly, i.e. there will therefore be a union between theory and practice, which facilitates the consolidation of information.

- *Materials used:* paper box, fancy paper, glue, personal hygiene items (toilet paper, flexi rods, toothbrush, toothpaste, soap, hand towel, shampoo, perfume, hair comb, nail scissors and others).

- Instructions: The first step is to cover the box with fancy paper, using glue. Afterwards, a hole should be made in the center of the box, which should be big enough for the children's hands to reach. Various hygiene objects should be placed inside the box. Each child will place one of their hands in the hole in the box, select a surprise object and then remove it from the box. Once this has been done, they will present the object to everyone present and answer the following questions: What is it, What is it for, How do I do it and Can I do it by myself?

Given the importance of the proposed theme, posters and/or pictures that deal with the topic can also be taken along, further reinforcing the issues of good habits with the children.

The formation of good health habits should be given special attention in this study, with the aim of consolidating appropriate habits already learned and acquiring new knowledge, attitudes and skills for healthy living. The child's attitudes towards good hygiene habits must be formed in such a way that, even if they lack the cooperation of the family, they persist and are later translated into behavior (NOVA EDIÇÂO PEDAGÒGICA PARA A ESCOLA MODERNA, 1989).

Therefore, it is believed that after this activity, the children will be given a greater share of responsibility for their daily routine in terms of health-related behavior, accompanying their development from dependence to independence.

6ª Stage: Sense organs

I Objectives

This new phase of the project focuses on the importance of making children aware of what the sense organs are, what they are used for and, above all, non-discrimination against people with disabilities.

The main function of these organs is to perceive what is happening around the individual, in other words, they bring "news" about the world around us (NEW PEDAGOGICAL EDITION FOR THE MODERN SCHOOL, 1989).

The sense of touch is located in the skin. It can be used to perceive cold, heat, pain and even the size and shape of objects. For children to understand this better, they should make correlations between certain situations and touch: "pain when you step on a nail", "perceiving the temperature of the water in the bath", "the pressure you feel when you hug", "feeling the softness of well-washed clothes", "the warmth of the sun" and "the coldness of ice cream" (NEW PEDAGOGICAL EDITION FOR THE MODERN SCHOOL, 1989).

The palate is a sense located on the tongue, thanks to which we can distinguish tastes: sour, sweet, bitter or salty. It is with it that we judge whether a juice has too much or too little sugar, whether a fruit is sweet or sour, whether food is salty or too little, or whether coffee is bitter (NOVA EDIÇÂO PEDAGÒGICA PARA A ESCOLA MODERNA, 1989).

The sense of smell is located in the nasal cavities (nose). When you use your sense of smell, you can perceive many things: the smell of a flower, chocolate, coffee, cooking gas, delicious food, garbage and many other things (NOVA EDIÇÂO PEDAGÒGICA PARA A ESCOLA MODERNA, 1989).

The eyes are responsible for vision. With this sense we can see people, objects, animals and many others (NOVA EDIÇÂO PEDAGÒGICA PARA A ESCOLA MODERNA, 1989).

Hearing is located in both ears. It is thanks to it that we perceive sounds: when someone calls us, when we hear music, birds singing, a car horn, a teacher's explanation and many other situations (NEW PEDAGOGICAL EDITION FOR THE MODERN SCHOOL, 1989).

II Dynamic activities

Here we will highlight two activities that aim to work with children on their sense organs: sight, taste, touch, smell and hearing.

1ª Activity: Sense game

- Materials used: a dark cloth, blindfolds, a pen, fruit, a toothbrush, toothpaste, dental floss, sugar, salt, a piece of bread, milk, cotton wool, sandpaper, a coin, a sponge, soap, perfume, vinegar, cinnamon, a rattle, crumpling paper.

- Instructions: The GAME OF SENSES will be played here. To do this, the class will be divided into five equal groups. Each group will have the name of a sense.

The name of each group and their number of correct answers will be written on the board. The group that gets the most objects right will win. This is how the game will be played:

Vision group:

Each member will be asked to look at the following material for one minute: pen, fruit, toothbrush, toothpaste and dental floss. Then cover these objects with a cloth, or blindfold the children, and ask each member of this group to say the name of all the objects they have seen - each correct answer justifies one point.

Taste group:

Blindfolded, one student at a time will try the following foods: sugar, salt, a piece of bread, fruit and milk. One point will be awarded for each food that is correct.

Touch group:

It's up to the group members to identify the following materials: cotton, sandpaper, coins, toothbrushes and sponges. As with the other groups, a point will be awarded for each correct answer.

Smell group:

Each student, with their eyes covered, will identify the following materials by smell: soap, fruit, perfume, vinegar and cinnamon. A point will be awarded for each correct answer.

Hearing group:

Each member of the group, blindfolded, will have to identify the following objects by sound: rattle, crumple paper, knock on the door, snap fingers and whistle. For each correct answer, a point will be awarded to the team.

2ª Activity: Toy telephone

- *Materials used:* string and disposable cups.
- Instructions: Make a hole in the bottom of each disposable cup. Then use a piece of string to connect the two cups. The toy telephone is another very interesting suggestion for working on the sense organs.

III Discussion

As has already been said, the aim here is to teach through play, but even playing requires learning, training and, above all, the training of our sense organs, which are responsible for training all the stimuli that surround us. According to Alves, p.20, 2005, *"our senses - sight, hearing, smell, touch, taste - are all organs for making love to the world, for taking pleasure in it".*

It is therefore believed that after carrying out these activities, the children will be able not only to receive stimuli, but also to interpret them. As a result, sensitive, critical and thinking individuals will be formed here - after all, thinking is an art.

7ª Stage: Food and nutrition

I Objectives

According to Angelis (2000), Anjos et al. (2003), Assis et al. (1999), Beighton et al. (1996), Birch (1999), Campos (2004), Chaves et al. (2000), Coury (2004), Governo de Minas Gerais (1999), Monteiro et al. (2003), Nóbrega (1998), Ramos et al. (2000), Sichieri et al. (2003), Tojo et al. and Vlitolo (2003) nutrition is one of the most important behavioral factors affecting the state of health of an individual or a nation. Therefore, the central axis of this stage will be familiarization and the commitment to raise awareness of the importance of good eating habits. So how, where and at what age is the best time to work on nutritional concepts?

How: through nutritional education, according to Nóbrega (1998), p. 42, "nutritional education is a subject of recognized importance". Continuing, the same author also states, p.42, that *"nutritional education should be integrated into Health Education programs, not restricted to transmitting concepts about nutrition and not interfering in the cultural process".*

With regard to the location, the school is one of the best places to work on this issue, since the children are at school for a long period of time, including a large part of their meals. In fact, if the school continues to turn a blind eye to this issue, classes will be divided between undernourished and obese pupils. Regarding the importance that the school environment can have on students' diets: if children don't eat well when they are at school, their dietary deficiencies can be supplemented with school meals (ANGELIS, 2000; ANJOS et al., 2003; ASSIS et al., 1999; BEIGHTON et al., 1996; BIRCH, 1999; CAMPOS, 2004; CHAVES et al., 2000; COURY, 2004; GOVERNO DE MINAS GERAIS, 1999; MONTEIRO et al., 2003; NÓBREGA, 1998; RAMOS et al., 2000; SICHIERI et al., 2003; TOJO et al. and VITOLO, 2003).

As for age, it is in childhood that eating habits are formed, making it necessary to understand their determining factors, so that it is possible to propose effective educational processes to change children's eating patterns (ASSIS et al., 1999; CAMPOS, 2004; CHAVES et al., 2000; COURY, 2004; TOJO et al. and VITOLO, 2003).

Angelis (2000), p. 47, defines malnutrition as *"any deviation from normal nutrition, either to a lesser degree, undernutrition, or to an excess, hypernutrition"*. It is a fact that an unbalanced diet poses great risks to people's health. Among the diseases resulting from inadequate eating habits are obesity, heart disease and tooth decay - widely known to be public health problems (ANGELIS, 2000; ANJOS et al., 2003; ASSIS et al., 1999; BEIGHTON et al., 1996; BIRCH, 1999; CAMPOS, 2004; CHAVES et al., 2000; COURY, 2004; GOVERNO DE MINAS GERAIS, 1999; MONTEIRO et al., 2003; NÓBREGA, 1998; RAMOS et al., 2000; SICHIERI et al., 2003; TOJO et al. and VITOLO, 2003).

According to Ramos and Stein (2000), p. 229, *"there is a consensus that changes in eating behavior are necessary to prevent food-related diseases and promote individual health"*.

Even so, food as health does not, in itself, represent a value for children - making it very difficult to get them to accept a varied diet. In order to do this, it is necessary to look for relationships between food and the purposes that are valuable to them, such as growth, physical vigor, attractive personal appearance, belonging to a group and having friends (BIRCH, 1999 and KOIVISTO, 1996).

It is in this context that the concept of promoting healthy eating practices also emerges, where a varied and balanced diet will be placed as one of the strategies for promoting health. After all, eating properly is very good for health, as each food has a different importance (RAMOS et al., 2000).

However, self-assessment of eating habits aims to develop in children, for whom independence is a very important value at this stage of life, a greater sense of responsibility for their own health at school (ANJOS et al., 2003; BIRCH, 1999; RAMOS et al., 2000; TOJO et al. and VITOLO, 2003).

The methodology, location and age range of this stage have been mentioned, but the definition and description of intelligent food consumption is still missing. In order to make this work easier and more didactic, posters and thematic illustrations should be produced.

Food is the nutritional substance ingested to replenish the energy, proteins, vitamins and minerals consumed by our body, in order to maintain physical and mental health (ANGELIS, 2000; COURY, 2004; N0BREGA, 1998).

In order to make it easier for people to understand the different types of food, a graphic way of distributing and grouping them has been sought: the food pyramid. It is common knowledge that a pyramid is a geometric figure with a larger base followed by a narrow apex, the importance of which lies in the subsequent description of the foods that follow. According to with Welsh (1992), p.12-23, the food pyramid was developed to ensure that various foods are consumed in sufficient quantities to make up a nutritionally adequate diet.

The food pyramid has been divided into four levels and illustrates the eight food groups (ANGELIS, 2000; COURY, 2004; NÓBREGA, 1998):

- At the first level of the pyramid, the base, is the group of cereals, pasta, tubers and roots. They should be consumed in greater quantities, as they provide all the daily energy needed by the body;
- The second level of the pyramid includes two groups, vegetables and fruit. Foods in this group are important for maintaining health because they offer fiber, vitamins and minerals;
- The third level includes three groups: milk and dairy products, meat and eggs and legumes. In this group, all foods are rich in the nutrient called protein and should be consumed in smaller quantities than the foods in the previous level;
- Finally, at the apex of the pyramid, there are two groups: oils and fats and sugars and sweets. These are rich in sugar, also known as simple carbohydrates. They should be consumed in smaller quantities than the other groups.

According to Philippi (1999) et al., p. 68, *"the eight groups were composed of similar foods and the number of servings per day for each group was defined"*. Each food group provides certain nutrients, but no group is more important than another. For the body to function properly, you need to include foods from all the groups in your diet.

We can therefore conclude that eating well is not about eating a lot, but about eating food that meets the needs of your body. It is better to value quality over quantity. To support a healthy diet, you should avoid too much salt, industrialized spices, animal fats and fried foods. We also recommend drinking filtered water, always washing your hands before meals and chewing your food well. These guidelines should be followed at all ages and throughout life (ANGELIS, 2000; ANJOS et al., 2003; ASSIS et al., 1999; BEIGHTON et al., 1996; BIRCH, 1999; CAMPOS, 2004; CHAVES et al.., 2000; COURY, 2004; GOVERNO DE MINAS GERAIS, 1999; MONTEIRO et al., 2003; NÓBREGA, 1998; RAMOS et al., 2000; SICHIERI et al., 2003; TOJO et al. and VITOLO, 2003).

II Dynamic activities

Four activities will be developed at this stage of the project, which will serve as strategies for working with the children in question on concepts relating to a balanced diet and, consequently, the benefits it brings. In this way, the students will be questioned and induced to be self-critical with the questions posed to them.

IªActivity: Getting to know the nutritionist through a story

Everyone knows how passionate children are about listening to stories. In fact, they're not satisfied with hearing them just once, they ask to hear them again and again. And just as important as listening to the stories is the children's participation in the narrative, the funny and clever things they say, and even the solutions they come up with for certain situations. Silva (1997), p. 10, states that *"the story makes everyone smile, the lesson becomes a fun game - and big people become children again"*. The author goes on to say, p. 12, *"the story calms, serenades, holds attention, informs, socializes, educates"*.

Finally, by using children's stories to raise questions about the importance of a proper diet, strategies for maintaining health are encouraged through make-believe play, provoking an imaginary situation that is at the same time governed by rules, encouraging the child to behave in a more advanced way than usual, acting directly on the child's behavioral changes.

- Materials used: creativity.

According to Silva, p. 13, 1997:

"the success of the narrative depends on several interconnected factors, and it is essential to draw up a plan, a script, in order to organize the narrator's performance, guaranteeing safety and ensuring naturalness."

- Instructions: Here we recommend that you first create characters. As you know, in a story there is usually a protagonist and an antagonist, who share a plot, a situation. In this situation, the protagonist will be the nutritionist - it is recommended to explain the professional's activity in detail, characterizing the benefits he or she will bring to the story and, consequently, to reality. In the case of the antagonist, you could create a fictional character, for example, "Dudu Bocâo", and relate in the story bad experiences that happened to this character who, because he eats too much and inappropriately, suffers from obesity, tooth decay, gastrointestinal discomfort, among others. The narrator should encourage the child to participate, to correlate the situations and, above all, to create solutions.

2ª Activity: Understanding the food pyramid

We mentioned earlier the importance of the food pyramid, which is a graphic representation that makes it easier to visualize foods and how to choose them for the day's meals (WELSH, 1992). It is therefore up to the children to clarify the food groups and their quantification, i.e. which foods should be eaten in greater quantities and which should be avoided - thus guaranteeing a balanced and, consequently, healthy diet.

- *Materials used:* cardboard, masking tape, illustrative food cut-outs.

- Instructions: Cut out the cardboard in a pyramidal shape. This pyramid should be divided into four levels: the first or base, a single cut, will represent the group of cereals, bread, tubers and roots; the second level should be divided into two pieces, one for the group of vegetables and the other for fruit; the third level will be divided into three parts, covering the groups of milk and milk products, meat and eggs and legumes; the fourth level or apex of the pyramid will include two groups, oils and fats and sugars and sweets, which should be consumed in moderation.After explaining how the food pyramid is divided, each child will be given a cut-out of some type of food. It will then be up to them to present the food and affix the figure to the food pyramid using masking tape.

3ªActivity: Assembling a healthy dish

After working through the theory, it's time to practice. Here we want to assess the children's ability to assemble a dish. This would characterize their learning in relation to the concepts passed on to them in relation to a balanced and healthy diet.

- *Materials used:* disposable plates and pictures of food (meal: lunch).

- Instructions: the children will set up a restaurant. The children are divided into groups, for example, the vitamin group, the vegetable group, the cereal group and so on. Each group will receive a plate on which they will assemble a meal, which in this case should be lunch. The group that puts together the dish most in line with a healthy diet will win.

4ªActivity: Making the fair

In this activity, the children will experience the sensation of being responsible for buying food, as well as working out how to control their money, since they will have a limit on their purchases. This will help them to discern what is necessary from what is superfluous when shopping.

- *Materials used:* fruit, bags, paper cut-outs symbolizing money (legal tender: FAZ-DE-CONTA, FDC$).

- Instructions: A fruit market will be set up in the school. All the food will be priced according to the current currency. The children will be divided into groups, each receiving a certain amount of money. This will be the day of the fruit salad, so the children will be responsible for buying the fruit, which will be brought in in bags provided for the students. Everyone should be aware that the same products will have different prices, so it's up to the groups to do some market research. So, as well as encouraging the children to get to know fruit, how it is arranged in the market and its importance for our health, the game here will also teach the students how to buy food.

We believe that at the end of these activities, students should appreciate a balanced diet and be able to relate it to quality of life.

8ª Step: Preventing domestic accidents

I Objectives

Addressing the prevention of health problems in the context of schools is part of the guidelines of public policies that established health education as a cross-cutting theme in Brazilian primary education. With this in mind, it is necessary to include these themes in the curricula of health professionals, since education is an important means of transforming and standardizing conducts that provide healthy environments, reducing the risk factors that exist within them. This partnership between education and health should help to reduce the accident rate, as well as raising awareness of the need to adopt preventive attitudes in the family, school and community. After all, safety is a health issue. The school has its share of responsibility for accident prevention and safety education (ALCÂNTARA et al., 2003; ARAÙJO et al., 2002; SOUZA et al., 2000; VIEIRA et al., 2005).

The literature focuses on the fact that education is considered one of the most important resources in accident prevention, and should be present in all programs with this purpose, included permanently in schools or other institutions, so that the educational process can take place. Schools are the ideal place to strengthen the implementation of preventive "seeds" in relation to accidents involving children and adolescents. Although most accidents involving children occur in the home, schools play a fundamental role in raising children's awareness the risks that permeate the home and the mechanisms for avoiding them (ALCÂNTARA et al., 2003; ARAÙJO et al., 2002; SOUZA et al., 2000; VIEIRA et al., 2005).

The home environment includes the physical structure, the behavior of the family and the daily activities that can, in certain situations, be a risk factor for domestic accidents. In the family context, children are more vulnerable to these accidents and families assume that they know the home environment very well, making them less vigilant and thus facilitating domestic accidents that have undesirable repercussions. It is necessary for the family, culturally considered to be responsible for promoting the safety and protection of its members, to become aware and be able to effectively carry out this preventive care (ALCÂNTARA et al., 2003; ARAÙJO et al., 2002; SOUZA et al., 2000; VIEIRA et al., 2005).

Strengthening the interaction between school and child, play is the moment we experience and remember from our childhood; associating preventive actions, simulations of cases using play as a reference is a possibility to be pursued in an attempt to minimize the occurrences of burns, falls, poisoning, aspiration of foreign bodies, physical aggression, among others that threaten the physical and social integrity of the little citizen. And this points to the fact that action in an imaginary situation teaches the child to direct their behavior not by the immediate perception of objects or the situation that affects them immediately, so it is impossible for the very young child to separate the field of meaning from the field of visual perception, since there is a very intimate fusion between Meaning and what is seen (ALCÂNTARA et al., 2003; ARAÙJO et al., 2002; SOUZA et al., 2000; VIEIRA et al., 2005).

This is the point in development when children can express their imagination, not only through language, but also through drawings, vocalizations and movements. Another premise is the need to stimulate the formation of "everyday" or "spontaneous" concepts that start from the child's practical activity and immediate social interactions (ALCÂNTARA et al., 2003; ARAÙJO et al., 2002; SOUZA et al., 2000; VIEIRA et al., 2005).

However, this stage aims to encourage children to take more responsibility for their own health, as they will be taught concepts aimed at a safe and healthy life.

II Dynamic activities

In order to encourage children to adopt healthy habits and reduce their risk of accidents, three activities will be carried out as part of this proposal.

1ª Activity: Meeting real heroes

What child hasn't dreamt of being a fireman, policeman or lifeguard? After all, these professionals are usually seen as heroes by them - which is true. So this activity will serve as a way of introducing these professionals to the children, in other words, they will get to know their heroes.

- Materials used: the presence of a policeman and a fireman.

- Instructions: on this day, a talk will be scheduled in advance with professionals who work directly with accident prevention or assistance. They could be police officers, members of the fire brigade or even volunteers, depending on the location. It will be up to the latter to explain and guide the children on what to do to avoid accidents and what to do when they happen.

2ª Activity: Play, learn and don't get hurt!

- *Materials used:* cut-outs of pictures depicting accidents.

- Instructions: the aim will be to collectively build resources that develop cognitive skills through the motor skills of cutting and pasting in the production of illustrated panels with educational messages. To do this, the children will be asked to bring in cut-outs on topics related to burns, animal bites, falls and collisions, electric shocks, injuries from sharp instruments, traffic accidents, among others. The pictures should be brought back by the school to make an illustrated panel on the proposed theme.

Activity 3: Providing help

A good way to consolidate concepts is by practicing them. So, this last activity will involve the children giving aid to a fictitious victim who has suffered an accident. As such, this dynamic will better equip those being assisted with the subject matter.

- *Materials used:* 01 telephone handset, 01 first aid kit (containing gauze, adhesive plaster and degermant) and 01 dummy.

- Instructions: Before preparing the game, the children should be told everything that is in a first aid kit and, above all, how to make a simple bandage. As well as the importance of staying calm in the event of an accident. And simple measures, such as the importance of washing wounds before applying bandages. The next step will be to set up the activity itself. With the help of a doll, the children will have to provide care for it. They will then have to bandage it. The children should also be taught how to call for help, with this focusing on the importance of knowing how to call the emergency room, the fire department and the police. This is where the telephone handset will be used to play the game.

III Discussion

Everyone has a responsibility to their community. Everyone can do many things for health, including providing help. With these activities, we believe that children will be made aware of a great attitude: to help. The help referred to here is not restricted to that given to potential victims, but mainly that given to the students: the ability to prevent accidents.

Second semester

9ª Step: Dentists and doctors are our friends

I Objectives

Society seems to have a negative image of dentists, and the dental experience is pre-judged as something that is almost always unpleasant and painful (AMORIM and SANTOS, 2000).

Children are often afraid of health professionals, especially dentists and doctors, due to false ideologies, whether created by the child themselves or induced by other people, usually their parents (AMORIM and SANTOS, 2000; ROSSETTI, 1999).

Therefore, it is essential that the dentist assesses the patient's perception of the dentist before any procedure, which can significantly influence the patient's reaction to dental treatment (AMORIM and SANTOS, 2000; ROSSETTI, 1999). Therefore, topics such as fear, white clothing, instruments used by the dental surgeon, surgical procedures and others should be addressed. The main aim of this phase is to dilute children's insecurity about health professionals.

II Dynamic activities

At this stage, two activities will be developed, the aim of which is to bring children closer to health professionals, especially dentists, who are usually insecure and fearful. The dynamics will be based on games, because the aim here is to play at being a dentist in order to like, or at least understand, this professional.

1ª Activity: Drawing the dentist

There are authors who have shown that through drawings children offer us various answers to childhood problems, many of which are difficult to express in any other way, such as verbally. Human figure drawings are therefore the richest source of information.

By drawing, the child uses an easy way to tell us their story at their level of understanding. Drawing is a way for children to express their fears, desires and fantasies. Through drawings, children communicate what is important to them and their concerns.

Drawing a human figure, in this case a specific person, the dentist, as a measure of attitude provides the child's feelings about this person. It is of the utmost importance to question the child about the drawing. This can give us additional information. It is important to remember that no drawing has meaning in isolation.

- *Materials used:* office paper, black pencil, eraser, colored pencils or felt-tip pens.

• <u>Instructions:</u> each child will be given a sheet of paper and their art materials and asked to draw the dentist. Once they have finished, each child will present their drawing, explaining it. This way, more data can be obtained to analyze the drawings.

2ª Activity: Who is a dentist anyway?

According to Salgado (2005) et al, p. 09:

"Thinking about children today requires a critical look at their increasingly complex social experiences. Living day after day with images, children and adults are weaving new experiences, ways of perceiving the world and themselves. Contemporary culture has images as its most intense form of expression".

In line with this line of thought, the aim here is to work with, or rather, to better educate those being treated about the real image they should have of the dental professional, whose aim is oral health and, consequently, a better quality of life for those who need it.

With this in mind, a good image of the dentist, the suggested activity is based on imitation and dramatization, since imitative and dramatized play allows the child to experience situations that are not those of their real life, but it is a way for them to give wings to their creative imagination, transforming situations presented to them and living them in a very real way (FAZIO, 2000; NOVA EDIÇÂO PEDAGÓGICA PARA A ESCOLA MODERNA, 1989; SILVA, 1997).

• <u>*Materials used:*</u> white clothing, stethoscope, sphygmomanometer, lab coat, mask, cap, goggles, procedure gloves, dental instruments, patient bib.

• <u>Instructions:</u> the activity consists of "assembling" a dentist. To do this, one of the members of this study must be dressed in white. From then on, the dentist will be introduced to the children, who will be asked about the possible professions that a person wearing white could have. The possible answers are awaited and then the children are asked if any of the professionals they have mentioned cause them fear. And if so, why. The aim of this stage is to show the children that they shouldn't be afraid of someone just because they're dressed in white - it's just a uniform - as these professionals are only looking out for our well-being. Afterwards, in order to interact with the world of health professionals, they will be shown all the items that belong to the uniform, such as the patient's coat, goggles, mask, cap, gloves and bib. They will also show the sphygmomanometer, the stethoscope and some dental instruments, which are usually the greatest cause of fear in patients.

III Discussion:

By carrying out these activities, the aim is to change, or rather shape, children's view of dentists through easy-to-play games. Perhaps after this stage we will one day see children "playing dentist", just as they have fun dressing up as policemen, firemen and other heroes they have created.

From this day onwards, it is recommended that all members of this study present themselves wearing white clothes and lab coats, reinforcing, or even offering, greater intimacy for these children with these uniforms.

10ª Step: Teeth and their functions

I Objectives

According to Martins (1999), p. 5-9, oral self-knowledge practices instituted in childhood can help build a new concept of oral health that stimulates self-esteem and, consequently, also motivates self-care actions, which are essential for full citizenship.

The main aim of this unit will be to give the children a better understanding of their teeth: they will be introduced to teeth, the different types of teeth and their functions, as well as how to care for them.

Teething is the formation and birth of teeth in the arches. During life, the deciduous teeth of childhood are gradually replaced by permanent teeth. This results in deciduous, mixed and permanent teeth (ARAÙJO, 1988; CORRÊA, 1998; OKESON, 2000).

The deciduous tooth, temporary tooth or milk tooth is the first tooth. It consists of twenty teeth, ten in each arch: 04 central incisors, 04 lateral incisors, 04 canines and 08 molars. These teeth are usually white in color, small and well separated from each other. Contrary to what many people think, these teeth have many functions, including chewing, speaking, guiding the eruption of permanent teeth, among others (ARAÙJO, 1988; CORRÊA, 1998; OKESON, 2000).

Mixed dentition is a transition between the first and second teeth. At this stage, the child has deciduous and permanent teeth at the same time. This phase begins with the appearance of the FIRST PERMANENT MOLARS. These teeth are of great importance, since they usually erupt at the age of six and should be quickly identified, since they are the teeth that remain in the oral cavity the longest and are therefore the most susceptible to caries (ARAÙJO, 1988; CORRÊA, 1998; OKESON, 2000).

The second or permanent tooth is the one that should remain in place for a person's entire life, which requires good hygiene and eating habits. It is made up of thirty-two teeth, eighteen in each arch: 04 central incisors, 04 lateral incisors, 04 canines, 08 premolars and 12 molars. The emergence of permanent teeth begins at the age of six and is completed around the age of eighteen with the third molars or wisdom teeth, which often don't even develop or don't have room for them in the arch. When compared to deciduous teeth, permanent teeth are larger, yellowish and have no spaces between them (ARAÙJO, 1988; CORRÊA, 1998; OKESON, 2000).

Just open your mouth and you can easily see that the teeth are different, both in terms of the shape of their crowns and their size. This is due to the different functions these teeth perform in chewing: the incisors have the function of grasping and cutting food. The canines pierce and tear food. The premolars crush food. The molars grind and crush food (ARAÙJO, 1988; CORRÊA, 1998; OKESON, 2000).

The importance of teeth in relation to food and nutrition should be emphasized here, as they are active instruments in preparing food for digestion.

With a little knowledge and by practicing simple care on a daily basis, you can have perfect, healthy teeth throughout your life. It's important to note that self-care is related to self-esteem, i.e. people who are stimulated and motivated dedicate themselves to practices that lead to health and well-being. In this way, this stage can become a valuable element in the search for oral health promotion.

II Dynamic activities

1ª Activity: Getting to know teeth and their functions

- *Materials used:* modeling clay, ruler and pencils.

- Instructions: each participant will be given a piece of modeling clay to model in the shape of a food that will be chewed - this is a great opportunity to reinforce the importance of healthy foods, so children should be encouraged to make models of fruit, vegetables and others. This activity aims to simulate the functions of the teeth. It starts with reproducing the function of the incisors. To do this, the dough should be cut with a ruler, which will simulate the incisors of these teeth. The next step will be to reproduce the action of the canines - with the tip of a pencil, the children will be asked to pierce the model already cut by the ruler. The last step will be for the children to take the fragments of food and place them in one of their hands, where they will crush them with great force, imitating the opening and closing movements of their mouths, as if they were grinding the food,

simulating the action of premolars and molars.

2ª Activity: Searching for the 1st permanent molar

- *Materials used:* cardboard, marker pens and/or colored pencils.
- Instructions: Make two illustrative posters, one representing deciduous dentition and the other mixed. Start by presenting the deciduous dentition, showing the children the teeth that make it up. Then, using a mixed dentition, draw all the deciduous teeth and the first permanent molar. It should be explained that these teeth appear around the age of six and do not replace any other teeth, but are located behind the deciduous second molar. With the help of a mirror, get the students to look at their teeth, assessing their number, color, position and so on.

III Discussion

The activities described here are aimed at motivating those assisted to carry out an oral self-examination, getting to know their teeth, their functions and how to care for them. This will make them more active and independent when it comes to their oral health. It will also serve as a method of assessing the condition of the students' teeth, reinforcing the importance of seeking advice from a dental surgeon if they have any doubts.

11ª Stage: Caries and periodontal disease

I Objectives

Of the diseases that affect the mouth, dental caries and periodontal diseases are the ones that occur most frequently in a large part of the population. The Brazilian population still has high rates of affected and lost teeth due to carious lesions and periodontal diseases, because they are unaware of the simplicity of prevention, or are unmotivated to practice it (AINAMO, 1989; ALONSO, 1990; *BATISTA, 2005;* CORRÊA, 1998; CARVALHO et al., 1999; CHIAPINOTTO, 2000; FERREIRA et al., 2004; TORRIANI, 1996).

The aim is to clarify the factors that cause these diseases, their consequences and, above all, how to prevent them.

The knowledge and attitudes of elementary school teachers regarding the etiology, development and prevention of dental caries and periodontal disease should be carefully assessed and, if necessary, revised, so that these educators can work together with the study team, contributing to the success of educational programs (SANTOS, 2002).

For these diseases to take hold, plaque must first be deposited, a whitish mass made up of food debris, oral fluids and microorganisms, which grows on the surface of the teeth. The type of bacterial colony is what differentiates the disease, i.e. whether it is tooth decay or periodontal disease. Therefore, removing plaque is a fundamental factor in preventing these diseases (AINAMO, 1989; ALONSO, 1990; *BATISTA, 2005;* CORRÊA, 1998; CARVALHO et al., 1999; CHIAPINOTTO, 2000; FERREIRA et al., 2004; TORRIANI, 1996).

> WORKING WITH CHILDREN ON CARIES

Students will be made aware that tooth decay is a disease, and like most diseases, it can be treated and, above all, prevented. This phase will take a longer period of time, as it will involve introducing concepts, raising awareness and changing habits.

The first step is to assess the level of knowledge of the assisted community regarding caries. After all, the implementation of the health education program must be carried out after the diagnosis of the target population, within the biopsychosocial context, not forgetting the family and cultural aspects in which they are inserted. This context permeates and influences the health issues and lifestyles of the community where the children live, making them a faithful portrait of their social reality and a reflection of the contradictions of the political and economic system the country is going through (ALVES *et al.*, 2004).

Second step: introducing concepts. Define the disease caries in a simplistic, clear and easy-to-understand, but not alienating, way (ASSOCIAÇÃO BRASILLERA DE ODoNToLoGiA, 2005):

"Dental caries is a communicable disease characterized by the loss of dental tissue due to demineralization and subsequent infection of these tissues. The plaque bacteria use the sugar consumed in our food in their metabolism, releasing acids that cause the demineralization of tooth enamel".

To make it easier for children to understand these concepts, the definition could be used like this: "a disease that causes "little holes" (cavities) in the teeth. It is caused by the "enemies of oral health", the so-called "caries bugs", which are also known as bacteria. In order to become "strong", these bacteria need to "feed", and their favorite food is sugar (found in candies, lollipops, chewing gum and sweets in general). After "eating" a lot, bacteria, just like people, have their "physiological needs" ("Pee" and "Poo"), which are eliminated in the mouth. The bacteria's "pee" and "poo" are called acids. And the latter attack destroying the teeth and can even lead to their "death" (loss) ".

Step three: treatment and prevention. Caries can only be treated by a dental surgeon, one of the greatest "friends of health". These professionals have "lethal weapons" that destroy all the "enemies" of oral health. Unlike treatment, which depends on the help of a professional, caries prevention can be carried out by anyone, regardless of age, gender or economic status, as it involves very simple measures: frequent and correct brushing, flossing, fluoridation and dietary changes.

> WORKING WITH CHILDREN ON PERIODONTAL DISEASE

It is a disease that affects the gums, the periodontal ligament and the alveolar bone, which are the structures that support the teeth in the arch. Therefore, it is also the cause of tooth loss (AINAMO, 1989; ASSOCIAÇÃO BRASILEIRA DE ODONTOLOGIA, 2005; coRRÊA, 1998; cHiAPiNoTTo, 2000; LAscALA et al., 1995; MARTiNs, 1999).

As with tooth decay, periodontal disease begins with the accumulation of bacterial plaque on the teeth and gums, which leads to an inflammatory condition that initially affects the gums (gingivitis) and, as the disease progresses, the supporting structures of the teeth (periodontitis) (AINAMO, 1989; ASSOCIAÇÃO BRAsILEIRA DE ODONTOLOGIA, 2005; cORRÊA, 1998; cHIAPINOTTO, 2000; LAScALA et al, 1995; MARTINS, 1999).

Periodontal disease should be treated by the dental surgeon. Removing plaque by brushing well and flossing is again the most effective method of prevention (AINAMO, 1989; ASSOcIAçÂO BRASILEIRA DE ODONTOLOGIA, 2005; cORRÊA, 1998; cHIAPINOTTO, 2000; LAScALA et al., 1995; MARTINS, 1999).

II Dynamic activities

1ª Activity: Identifying bacterial plaque

- *Materials used:* cardboard, suede paper or paper towels, scissors, glue, colored pencils and/or felt-tip pens.
- Instructions: Draw a smiley face on the cardboard, using colored pencils and felt-tip pens. Cut out the suede paper in the shape of some teeth, which should be glued onto the smile. This will leave some teeth smooth and others rough. The children should be shown the smile and then explained that the teeth that have plaque on them will have an altered, rough texture. Ask the children to run their hands over their teeth and find the ones that have been brushed badly. Afterwards, explain to the children that the same thing happens to them - just run your tongue over your teeth before and after brushing and notice the difference in their smoothness.

2nd Activity: How the flu happens

- *Materials used:* office paper, suede paper or towel, coffee powder, colored pencils and/or felt-tip pens, scissors.
- Instructions: two teeth will be cut out, one on official paper and one on a paper towel.

On the paper tooth you draw an expression of happiness, while on the paper towel you draw a sad face. Afterwards, show the children the paper tooth, which is happy because it is smooth and clean - due to proper hygiene and nutrition. On the other hand, when the teeth are poorly cared for, they will look like the paper towel teeth, rough and sad. The two paper teeth should be handled by each child so that they can feel the difference in texture. The next step will be to prove that the rough tooth has plaque, through an experiment. To prove this, coffee powder will be used, which should be stored in a jar - the children will be told that there are "caries bugs" stored there. Rub a little coffee powder on both teeth, paper and towel. Once this step is complete, simply lift the teeth and wait for the result: on the smooth, paper tooth, all the powder will fall to the ground, confirming that this tooth is free of plaque and of cavities and periodontal disease; on the paper towel tooth, the coffee powder will be trapped when the paper is lifted, thus confirming the presence of plaque and the risk of this tooth acquiring the aforementioned diseases.

3ª Activity: Exploding the cavity

- *Materials used:* white balloons, office paper, marker pens, scissors and masking tape.
- Instructions: five caries "animals" and eleven smiles will be drawn on official paper, cut out and then stuck to the white balloons filled with air using masking tape. It's important that they are odd numbers, to avoid the risk of a tie. In fact, the balloons act as teeth, i.e. the ones that are smiling correspond to healthy teeth, while the others represent teeth attacked by decay. To play the game, the class will be divided into two groups (Brush Class and Floss Class). The rules of the game are that each participant takes one balloon at a time and has to pop it on the wall. However, they have to choose the right balloon because they have to keep the sticker on it. The class that pops the most decayed teeth will be the losers and the class that brings the most healthy teeth will win the game.

III Discussion

Of course, the construction of oral health as a value is associated with the conquest of social rights, decent living conditions, work, housing and access to good quality health services. However, these activities are not intended to solve the oral health problem once and for all, but they do aim to provide guidance to those being treated about its existence and, above all, its prevention, using a dynamic and fun methodology.

12ª Step: Toothbrush

I Objectives

Brushing, when done properly, is the most effective way of preventing the onset of diseases that affect the oral cavity, especially tooth decay and periodontal disease. The toothbrush is the most widely used and socially accepted instrument of oral hygiene, so to ensure its effectiveness during brushing, it must be taught and motivated (ALVES et al., 2003; BARRA et al., 1990; FIGUEIREDO et al., 1990).

At this stage, the project team will have to pay attention to the quantity and quality of toothbrushes used by the children. A "toothbrush bank" should be organized at the school, where the children would be registered to receive new toothbrushes, either because they don't have one or because they need to change. Toothbrushes can be requested from parents or obtained through donations, proposing partnerships with public bodies, such as the City Hall, and/or private organizations.

II Dynamic activities

1ª Activity: My toothbrush looks like this

- Materials used: a large bath brush.
- Instructions: using a large bath brush, the members of the project will present and describe the parts of the brush: the handle; the rod that connects the handle to the brush head; the head; the bristles, which must be firm to guarantee the brush's hygienic function; if the tufts are turned or bent the brush needs to be replaced.

It is necessary for each child to have their own toothbrush in hand, as they will be stimulated by the lecture and will learn more.

2ª Activity: Making the eco-brush

- Materials used: vegetable loofah, bamboo or wooden stick and string or thread 10.
- Instructions: with the aim of devising a toothbrush that would be effective for oral hygiene and at the same time affordable for the poor, Barra and Lima (1990) presented the ecological toothbrush. The study was carried out with the aim of comparing the amount of plaque removed by the eco-brush and the conventional toothbrush. The authors concluded that there was no difference in the amount of plaque removed by the brushes used, and that the eco-brush can be used as an alternative and economical means of oral hygiene. To make it: use a wooden or bamboo stick to attach the vegetable loofah using string or 10 thread. The brush should be used like an industrial toothbrush, i.e. to brush your teeth after meals.

It is believed that after carrying out these activities, the children will not only be familiar with the toothbrush, but will also feel motivated to use it, since it plays an active role in removing plaque and, consequently, in preventing cavities and periodontal diseases.

13ª Step: Toothpaste and floss

I Objectives

Toothpastes help to make brushing more pleasant, in addition to their bactericidal action and fluoride supplementation. Currently in Brazil, all toothpastes are fluoridated, which means that some precautions should be taken regarding the age and/or inability of children to control expectoration, as well as assessing whether there is another systemic route of fluoride.

Fluoride toothpaste should be used with caution, contrary to what is normally done, the amount of toothpaste needed for brushing is small, to avoid excess product, it is recommended to place it on the brush in a transverse direction - contrary to what is seen in the media, where a large amount of toothpaste is placed (ARMONIA et al., 1998 and BITTENCOURT et al., 1998 and CORRÊA, 1998 and FELDENS et al., 2001 and HOLLOWAY et al., 1997 and LEVY et al., 1995 and LIMA et al., 2001 and MOTTA et al., 2002 and SECRETARIA DE SAÙDE, 2000 and SERRA, 1992 and TORRIANI 1996).

As mentioned, brushing alone does not completely remove biofilm from tooth surfaces. The greatest difficulty lies in the interproximal region, where removal by brushing alone is deficient. For this reason, dental floss is considered a highly effective device to supplement brushing. Flossing is important for removing biofilm in the interproximal region, as this is where tooth decay and periodontal disease are usually most severe (ALVES, 2003; COSTA, 1996). Children should be taught that flossing should be done with the assistance of an adult, as they could end up cutting oral tissues.

II Dynamic activities

1ª Activity: Presentation of floss and toothpaste

- Materials used: toothbrush, toothpaste, dental floss, fancy paper, two white plastic cups and adhesive tape.
- Instructions (Toothpaste): with a box of toothpaste, the speaker should begin the presentation of the product: first, the packaging should be shown, which provides the consumer with some important information, including the expiry date, the presence or absence of fluoride, as well as the indication of the product. The next step is to present the toothpaste tube, which should always be closed to prevent the product from drying out. Demonstrate how to use the toothpaste, which should be applied in small quantities to the

toothbrush, as too much could make it easier to swallow. It is recommended that the project members demonstrate to everyone present how much paste should be put on the toothbrush. Warn the children that the only utensil that should be associated with the use of toothpaste is the toothbrush, since some people use fingers to brush, which is not only ineffective, but can also bring microorganisms into the oral cavity.

- Instructions (dental floss): two white plastic cups should be attached to each other using adhesive tape - simulating proximal contact between two neighboring teeth. In addition, small geometric figures should be cut out of fantasy paper and glued onto the cups to represent food debris adhered to the teeth. Present the diagram of the proximal contacts made with the plastic cups. Explain that there is a space between two teeth that is not reached by the toothbrush, the interdental space, and that this space, when not properly cleaned , is responsible for a high incidence of carious lesions. This is easily explained by adapting the geometric figures previously cut out on all the faces of the schematic model, since the toothbrush would be able to remove all the figures except those on the interproximal faces. To achieve this, interdental hygiene, it would be necessary to use dental floss. Present the packaging, the amount of floss to be cut and how to use it. Once this is done, the floss should be demonstrated on the schematic model, i.e. the removal of the figures stuck between the two glasses, simulating the function of the floss in interdental hygiene.

2ª Activity: Learning to make dental tape

- Materials used: plastic packaging bag

- Instructions: due to the socio-economic differences that affect a large part of the population, it is difficult to buy dental floss, which is often seen as something superfluous. Therefore, children will be taught how to make an interdental tape, looking for alternative means of interdental hygiene. All they have to do to make this tape is cut plastic bags into strips and then perform interdental hygiene. In relation to the efficiency of removing bacterial biofilm in the interproximal region by these alternative dental strips, the study by Costa and Corrêa (1996) found that this device removed biofilm in the same proportion as conventional dental floss, and could be indicated as an alternative to supplement brushing.

3rd Activity: Memory game.

- Materials used: cardboard, illustrative figures, felt-tip pens and/or colored pencils.

- Instructions: the game should be handmade with cardboard and illustrative figures (smiling tooth, toothbrush, dental floss, toothpaste and "caries bug" - all in pairs). The first step will be to glue the pictures onto the cardboard and then cut them out - making a memory game. The rules are very simple: first, place the cards face down and ask the players to form pairs.

The winner of the game will be whoever forms the most pairs and the loser will be whoever forms the fewest. In addition, whoever forms two pairs of the cards that offer the "caries bug" as a face will be disqualified.

III Discussion

One of the main objectives of this stage is to make the patients aware of the need to control bacterial biofilm and, consequently, prevent tooth decay and periodontal diseases. It's not just about knowing how to use a toothbrush, toothpaste and dental floss, but also how to use them, using systematized techniques.

<u>14ª Step: Brushing my teeth</u>

I Objectives

Oral hygiene is a fundamental component of people's body hygiene. But performing it properly requires learning. One of the possibilities for this learning is the development of supervised oral hygiene activities, adapting hygiene to the individual's motor skills. Caution is recommended when defining "correct" and "wrong" techniques, to avoid stigmatization.

Therefore, after introducing the toothbrush, toothpaste and dental floss, this is the ideal time to teach, correct and even reinforce the importance of how to properly clean the oral cavity. The main objective is to ensure that the teeth are properly cleaned, and this requires time and technique, since the lack of these would lead to poor hygiene. The aim here is to encourage children to brush independently. It will be up to the members of the project to make brushing a pleasurable experience, since it is self-care. According to Coury (2004), p. 257, *"self-care is essential to complete any treatment and to prevent diseases"*.

II Dynamic activities:

1ª Activity: Learning to brush my teeth

- <u>Materials used:</u> dental mannequin, toothbrush, dentifrice and dental floss.
- <u>Instructions:</u> the children will be divided into groups and each group will be assisted by a member of the project, who will reproduce everything that the central speaker will do. First, the children will be shown the dental mannequins, where it will be explained to them that this is a representation of the oral cavity and that it will be very helpful in teaching them how to brush, which follows an execution plan. After the mannequins have been presented, they

will start brushing their teeth. The children will be shown an analogy between cleaning the oral cavity and cleaning a "house", since it has several "windows", the teeth, and a floor that must be very clean, the tongue. Tell the children that they should take care of their teeth like they take care of their own house, making sure both are clean and smell good. With the toothbrush loaded with toothpaste, slightly tilted and resting against the gums, try to clean every two teeth, using circular and gentle movements ("balls"). You should start with the molars of the upper arch on the outer left until you reach the molars on the outer right. Then, on these last teeth, the upper right molars, the face is changed, i.e. the brushing is moved to the inner side, until it reaches the inner faces of the upper left molars. The occlusal surfaces of the posterior teeth will be brushed with back-and-forth movements. Friction movements ("chuveirinho") will be applied to the anterior teeth to optimize cleaning. All these processes should also be carried out on the lower arch. To complete the brushing, the tongue should be brushed from the inside out, and dental floss should be used to ensure interproximal hygiene (ARAÙJO, 1988; ASSOCIAÇÃO BRASILEIRA DE ODONTOLOGIA, 2005; CORREA, 1998; CURY, 1999).

2ª Activity: Supervised brushing

- Materials used: toothbrush, toothpaste, dental floss and dental students to supervise brushing.

- Instructions: the previously taught practice will be carried out. Brushing techniques will be evaluated, as well as the need for corrections and improvements. Brushing will be done after the children have eaten. All aspects of brushing should be observed: the amount of toothpaste used by the child, how the child holds the toothbrush, brushing movements, tongue cleaning, flossing, mouth rinsing and even water wastage during brushing, since this natural resource is exhaustible and of paramount importance for people's comfort and health.

The conclusion is that carrying out this stage instills in the children not only the importance of brushing, but also the concern to do it correctly. In addition, these activities aim to motivate the children, offering them not only concepts, but also making them active and participative in the actions that affect their health, combining education and health with moments of pleasure and joy.

15ª Step: Plaque developer and fluorine

I Objectives

> THE PLATE DEVELOPER

The so-called bacterial plaque is a film that is invisible to the naked eye. To identify it, there are substances that dye it: plaque developer, a chemical agent that has the function of identifying the presence or not of bacterial plaque, as well as serving as a vehicle collaborating with oral hygiene, since it is able to identify areas that are being less favored with poor brushing (ARAÙJO, 1988; ASSOCIAÇÃO BRASILEIRA DE ODONTOLOGIA, 2005; CORREA, 1998; CURY, 1999; SILVA, 1999).

A common example is the 2% hydroalcoholic substance fuchsin basica applied topically. In order to avoid staining soft tissue, basic fuchsin is applied directly to the tooth surface with a flexible rod or brush. The excess dye is then removed with a jet of water and the stained surfaces, which represent areas where brushing is not reaching or is ineffective, are quantified immediately afterwards (ARAÙJO, 1988; ASSOCIAÇÃO BRASILEIRA DE ODONTOLOGIA, 2005; CORREA, 1998; CURY, 1999; SILVA,).

The plaque developer should be presented to the children as a "magic liquid" capable of showing where the tooth decay "bug" is "living". However, it would facilitate the action of motivating those being assisted, since it locates the "enemy", for further "combat": hygienization.

> THE FLOWER

The main objective here will be to introduce fluorine, which will also be referred to as the "friend of health". Fluorine is a chemical element that participates in the formation of teeth and bones (ARAÙJO, 1988; ASSOCIAÇÃO BRASILEIRA DE ODONTOLOGIA, 2005; CORRÊA, 1998; CURY, 1999; SILVA, 1999). For children, a "magic substance" capable of making their teeth "stronger" and, consequently, healthier.

Typical fluoride application agents have been tested since the 1940s. Initially, their function in the preventive context was considered secondary. However, nowadays, after evaluating the significant decline in the incidence of dental caries observed over the last two decades in developed countries, they are no longer underestimated and have come to occupy an important place in therapeutic/preventive programs for dental caries (ARAÙJO, 1988; ASSOCIAÇÃO BRASILEIRA DE ODONTOLOGIA, 2005; CORRÊA, 1998; CURY, 1999; SILVA, 1999).

Today there are various forms of typical use of fluoride compounds available, including: fluoride toothpastes, fluoride varnishes, fluoridated water and fluoride gels. Fluoride gels are used according to each individual's needs, so their use should always be supervised by a dental surgeon. Ingesting large quantities of fluoride is toxic to the body (ASSOCIAÇÃO

BRASILEIRA DE ODONTOLOGIA, 2005 and CORRÊA, 1998 and CRUZ, 1999 and TORRIANI, 1996).

II Dynamic activities

Activity: Typical application of plate and fluoride developer

- Materials used: fluoride gel, plaque developer, flexible rods, toothbrush, dentifrice, dental floss and dental students to supervise brushing.

- Instructions: the activity will begin with supervised brushing, so in order to ensure optimum prophylaxis for the children, plaque developer should be applied to them with the flexible rods and, with the help of a mirror, the children should be made aware of the stained surfaces and regions - where brushing is deficient, reinforcing the importance of supplementing it. As for the fluoride application technique, some recommendations should be followed: prior prophylaxis, application time (four minutes) and instructions not to rinse the oral cavity, drink or eat food during the subsequent 30 minutes have been indicated and adhered to since the beginning of its use (ARAÙJO, 1988; ASSOCIAÇÂO BRASILEIRA DE ODONTOLOGIA, 2005; CORRÊA, 1998; CURY, 1999; SILVA, 1999).

III Discussion

This activity is described in its context as a collective intervention in oral health. It aims to reach the people it assists through collective actions, popularizing preventive concepts. After all, one of the functions of the dentist, which is usually forgotten, is to educate, in this case, to educate in health.

16ª Stage: Closing

It is known that the success of a project is its continuity, but this responsibility should be passed on to those who are directly involved in caring for the children: parents and/or guardians and the school staff. In order to raise their awareness, a talk should be scheduled with them. The members of the project will have to cover various topics, including: the aims of the project; the importance of preventive methods and their effectiveness against various diseases; the definition, etiology and preventive methods of caries and periodontal diseases; toothbrushes, dental floss, dentifrices and their use; teeth; the importance of diet; the importance of the family, the questionnaires administered to the children and family, among others. In addition to the conceptual presentation, the members of the project should be able to solve any questions that may be raised by those present at the meeting in a simple and effective way. After all, communication is the basis for any satisfactory relationship, and it is a key point for the interaction between dentist/child and dentist/parents.

At the end of the meeting, there will also be a farewell with the children, which will be attended by all the members of the project. On this day, each child will also receive a card **(Annex),** which attests to their responsibility for a healthy life, since at that moment they will have just been consecrated as a **"HEALTH WARRIOR".** In addition to the card, certificates will also be awarded

(Annex) for each classroom, showing that everyone in that school is defending people's health and well-being.

The conclusion is that after this project was carried out, not only was the issue of oral health addressed, but the citizenship of all those assisted was also rescued. After all, it is a child's right to have an education, to be healthy and, above all, to play.

Final considerations

It can be concluded that the proposed Educational Program:

- It has simple, low-cost educational and motivational strategies that can be applied in different socio-educational environments and is compatible with the Brazilian reality;
- It allows exchanges between the university and the community, enabling academics to participate more actively with the population;
- It aims to provide schoolchildren with a better level of knowledge about general and oral health, while still offering them a moment of leisure, i.e. combining education with pleasure;
- It seeks to make the children it serves carriers of knowledge for the subsequent education of young people and adults;
- It aims to make everyone aware of the importance of preventive methods;
- It aims to work with educators, who must re-evaluate their concepts and become aware of the responsibility they have over their students in terms of practicing healthy habits;
- It aims to improve the relationship between schoolchildren and health professionals;
- Demystifying inadequate beliefs, attitudes and behaviors in relation to health;
- Promoting physical and mental health for all those served.

Only through a commitment to health education, in the pursuit of preventive care, will we be able to offer everyone a better vision of their rights, as well as awareness of their real role as agents of their own health. This will effectively lead to a better standard of living for the entire population.

Bibliographical references

1. AINAMO, J. Epidemiology of Periodontal Disease. In: LINDHE, J. **Tratado de Periodontologia Clinica**. 2ª edição. Rio de Janeiro: Editora Guanabara Koogan. p. 42-57. 1989.

2. ALCÂNTARA, D. A,; VIEIRA L. J. E. S.; ALBUQUERQUE V. L. M. Drug poisoning in children. **Revista Brasileira em Promoçâo da Saù**. I6:10-6. 2003.

ALMEIDA, P. N. **Educaçâo Lúdica / Técnicas e jogos pedagógicos**. 6th edition. Sâo Paulo: Ediçôes Loyola. p. 15-22. 1994.

3. ALONSO, M. E. A. **Current situation of social dentistry teaching in three selected higher education institutions in the state of Rio de Janeiro**. Dissertation (Master's degree in social dentistry). Fluminense Federal University, Rio de Janeiro. 79 p. 1990.

4. ALVES, D. M. et al. Evaluation of the effectiveness of an alternative toothbrush and tape in oral hygiene in public school children. **Rev. Odontologia Clin.-Cientif**. 2(3): p. 191195. 2003.

5. ALVES, M. U.; VOLSCHAN, B. C. G.; HASS, N. A. T. Oral health education: sensitization of parents of children treated at the integrated clinic of two private universities. Pesq. Bras. **Odontoped. Clin. Integr**. Joâo Pessoa, 4(1): p. 47-51.2004.

6. ALVES, R. **Education of the senses and more...** / Rubem Alves. Campinas, SP: Verus Editora. 126 p. 2005.

7. AMARAL, M. C. P. **Perfil de cirurgiâo: dentista do serviço público do município do Rio de Janeiro**. Dissertation (Master's Degree in Social Dentistry). Fluminense Federal University, Rio de Janeiro. 105 p. 1991.

8. AMORIM, V. C. S. A.; SANTOS, M. F. S. Children's vision of the dentist through the interpretation of drawings. **Rev. ABO Nac**. 7(6): 359-363. 2000.

9. ANGELIS, R. C. **Hidden hunger: Physiological bases for reducing your risks through healthy eating**. Sâo Paulo: Editora Atheneu. p. 3-4, 47, 79, 112-115, 123, 133-138, 161-164, 177-178, 188-195, 206-216, 222-223. 2000.

10. ANJOS, L. A. et al. Growth and nutritional status in a probabilistic sample of schoolchildren in the Municipality of Rio de Janeiro. **Cadernos de Saùblica**. 19(1): 171-179. 2003.

11. AQUILANTE, A. G. et al. The importance of oral health education for preschoolers.

Revista de Odontologia da UNESP. Sâo Paulo. 32 (1): p. 39-45. 2003.

12. ARAÙJO, K. L,; VIEIRA L. J. E. S. Children and risk factors in the home and school environment: a reflective essay. **Texto Contexto Enferm**. 11(3): 83-7. 2002.

13. ARAÙJO, M. C. M. **Orthodontics for clinicians**. 4ªedition. Sâo Paulo: Editora Santos. Chap. 2,3. p. 27-96. 1988.

14. ARMONIA, P. L. et al. Risks of dental fluorosis in three-year-old children living in the municipality of São Paulo who use fluoridated toothpaste. **Rev. Inst. Ciênc. Saùde**. 16(1): 13-19. 1998.

15. ASSIS, M. A. A.; NAHAS, M. V. Aspectos motivacionais em programas de mudança de comportamento alimentar. **Rev. Nutr. PUCCAMP**. 12(1): p. 33-41. 1999.

16. BRAZILIAN DENTAL ASSOCIATION - RIO DE JANEIRO SECTION. **Training course for Community Oral Health Agents**. Department of Community Activities. 2005.

17. BARATA, R. B. et al. Condiçôes de vida e situaçao de saù. Saùde Movimento, 4. Abrasco. Rio de Janeiro, Baussel R. B. Quality-of-life assessment in outcomes research. **Evaluation & The Health Professions**. 21 (2): 139-140. 1997.

18. BARRA, R. P.; LIMA, T. B. F. Ecological toothbrush: an alternative for plaque removal. **Revista Cientifica Ciências Biomédica da Universidade Federal de Uberlândia**. 6: 24-27. 1990.

19. BARRoS, A. J. D. **Health Risks among Child Day Care Center Attendees: The Role of Day Care Centre Characteristics in Common Childhood Illnesses**. Ph.D. Thesis, London: London School of Hygiene and Tropical Medicine, University of London. 1996.

20. BATISTA, R. M. Health education for dental professionals and the population, a path to participation and improved health. **Medcenter: Social and preventive dentistry**. Article. Published December 7, 2005. Accessed on January 21, 2006. Available at< http://www.odontologia.com.br/artigos.asp?id=597&idesp=12&ler=s>. 2005.

21. BEIGHToN, D.; ADAMSoN, A.; RUGG-GUNN, A. Associations between dietary intake, dental caries experience and salivary bacterial levels in 12-year-old English schoolchildren. **Archs oral Biol**. 41(3): 271-280. 1996.

22. BITTENCOURT, L. P. et al. Identification of risk factors for fluorosis - a case report. **JBP.** 1(4): 17-23. 1998.

23. BOLIVAR, A. The school as a learning organization. In: CANARIO, Rui. (Org.). **Training**

and work situations. Porto: Porto Editora. p. 79-100. 1997.

24. BRAZIL. SECRETARIAT OF FUNDAMENTAL EDUCATION. **Paramétras Curriculares nacionais: terceiro e quarto ciclos: apresentaçâo dos temas transversais** / Secretaria de Educaçâo Fundamental. Brasilia: MEC/SEF. p-247-265. 1998.

25. BRAZIL 1999. **Saùde da familia no Brasil: linhas estratégicas para o quadriênio 1999/2002**. Ministry of Health, Brasilia. 1999.

26. BERGE, A. **Como educar pais e filhos?** / Faculdade de Educaçâo - Coleçâo Familia 1; translation: Tereza de Araùjo Penna. Rio de Janeiro: Livraria Agir Editora. p. 19-48. 1968.

27. BIRCH, L. L. **The patterns of food acceptance by children**. Nestlé Annals. 57: 1220. 1999.

28. BRITO BASTOS, N. C. Educaçâo para a Saù na Escola. **FSESP Magazine**. 9 (2). 1979.

29. BROUGÉRE, G. Jogo e Educaçâo: Traduçâo Patricia Chinotti Ramos. Porto Alegre, **RGS: Artes Médicas**. p. 43. 1998.

30. BUSS, P. M. Health promotion and education at the School of Government in Health of the National School of Public Health. **Cad Saùde Pùblica**. 15(2):177-85. 1999.

31. CABRAL,T. C. T. Motivation: the great challenge. **Revista Fluminense de Saùde Coletiva**. Niterói. 1 (4): p 23-32. 1998.

32. CADERNOS DE EDUCAÇÃO POPULAR 7. **Health and popular education**. Organized by Nova - Pesquisa, Assessoramento e Avaliaçâo em Educaçâo. The question of health and illness. Petrópolis: Editora Vozes. p.43-47. 1984.

33. CAMPOS, J. A. D. B. School meals and health promotion. **Rev. Cienc. Odontol. Bras**. 7(3): 67-71. 2004.

34. CANGUSSU, M. C. T.; MAGNAVITA, R.; ROCHA, M. C. B. S. Education and citizenship building in an oral health program in Salvador - BA.

Aboprev Magazine - Living in health. Salvador, 4 (1): 15-20. 2001.

35. CARVALHO, I. M. M.; ALMEIDA, P. H. **Familia e proteçâo social**. Sâo Paulo Perspec. [online]. abr./jun. 2003, vol.17, no.2 [cited 28 January 2006], p.109-122. Available at World Wide Web: <http://www.scielo.br/scielo.php?script=sci_arttext&pid=S0102-88392003000200012&lng=en&nrm=iso>. ISSN 0102-8839. 2003.

36. CARVALHO, J.; MALTZ M. Oral health promotion: Aboprev. **Diagnosis of caries**. In: Kriger, L.. Sâo Paulo: Editora Artes Médicas. p. 69-91. 1999.

37. CAVALLARI, V. R.; ZACHARIAS, V. **Trabalhando com recreaçâo**. 2ª edição. Sâo Paulo: Editora icone. 13-20; 55-65. 1994.

38. CHÂTEAU, J. **O jogo e a criança** / Jean Chateau; traduçâo: Guido de Almeida. Sâo Paulo: Summus. p. 13-33; 125-137. 1987.

39. CHAVES, S. C. et al. The effectiveness of preventive actions in controlling dental caries among schoolchildren: a comparison between two groups. **Revista da ABOPREV**. 3(2): 57-64. 2000.

40. CHIAPINOTTO, G. A. Collective Oral Health. In: PINTO, V. G. **Etiologia e Prevençâo da Doença Periodontal**. Sâo Paulo: Editora Santos. p. 429-444. 2000.

41. COLLARES, C. A. L.; MOISÉS M. A. A. Educaçâo , Saù e Formaçâo da Cidadania. **Education and Society**. Sâo Paulo. 10 (32). 1989.

42. REGIONAL COUNCIL OF NUTRITIONISTS. Interdisciplinarity: the various professional approaches are given a single language and the patient is seen in their own particular way. **Revista CRN**.1(1): p. 8-11. 2006.

43. CORRÊA, M. S. N. O. **Pediatric Dentistry in Early Childhood**. 1st Edition. Sâo Paulo: Editora e Livraria Santos. p. 206; 271-78; 315-342; 169;181. 1998.

44. COSTA, A. F.; CORREA, D. L.; CORREA, V. C. Alternative floss substitutes.

Paraense Journal of Dentistry. 1: 9-12. 1996.

45. COSTA I. C. C.; ALBUQUERQUE, A. J. **Health education**. In: Preventive and social dentistry: selected texts. Natal: EDUFRN. p. 223-50. 1997.

46. COURY, S. T. **Vital nutrition: a holistic approach to food and health**.

Brasilia: LGE Editora. p. 26-29, 40, 102-105, 253-264. 2004.

47. CRUZ, R. A. **Clinical and laboratory considerations on the reactivity of fluoride compounds applied topically to human dental enamel**. In: KRIGER, L. Promoçâo de Saúde Bucal: ABOPREV. 2nd edition. Sâo Paulo: Artes Médicas. p. 167-194. 1999.

48. CURY, J. A. **Mechanical control of dental plaque by the patient**. In: KRIGER, L. Promoçâo de Saúde Bucal: ABOPREV. 2nd edition. Sâo Paulo: Artes Médicas. p.113-128. 1999.

49. CURY, J. A. **Chemical control of dental plaque**. In: KRIGER, L. Promoçâo de Saúde Bucal: ABOPREV. 2nd edition. Sâo Paulo: Artes Médicas. p.129-140. 1999.

DUARTE JR, J. F. Why art education? 3ª edition. Campinas: Papirus. p.67. 1995.

50. FAZIO, L. S. Storytelling, inventing stories and fantasy recreation. In: Parham, L. D., Fazio LS. **Recreation in pediatric occupational therapy**. Sâo Paulo: Santos. p.233-47. 2000.

51. FELDENS, E. G. et al. Evaluation of the use of fluoride dentifrices by children aged 2 to 5 years from three schools in the city of Porto Alegre. **JBP**. 4(21): 376-382. 2001.

52. FERREIRA, R. I. et al. Oral health education for adult patients: Report of an experience. **Revista de Odontologia da UNESP**. 33(3): p. 149-155. 2004.

53. FIGUEIREDO, M. C.; BELLO, D. Comparative evaluation of the effectiveness of an alternative toothbrush and a conventional toothbrush in removing dental plaque. **Revista da Faculdade de Odontologia Universidade de Passo Fundo**. 4: 13-20. 1999.

54. FREIRE, J. B. **Full-body education**. Sâo Paulo: Scipione. p. 13. 1989.

55. FREIRE, J. B. Before talking about Motor Education. In: DE MARCO, Ademir (org). **Thinking about Motor Education**. Sâo Paulo: Papirus. p. 43. 1995.

56. FIGUEIREDO, R. V. Inclusion policies: school-management of learning in diversity. In ROSA, E. G. and SOUZA, V. C. **Politicas organizativas e curriculares, educaçâo inclusiva e formaçâo de professores**. Rio de Janeiro: DP&A Editora. p. 68. 2002.

57. FORTUNA, T. R. Training teachers to play at university. In: SANTOS, S. M. P. **A ludicidade como ciência**. Petrópolis: Vozes. p.116. 2001.

58. GARCIA, P. P. N. S. et al. Oral Health Knowledge in Schoolchildren: Effect of a Self-Instruction Method. **Revista de Odontologia da UNESP**. Sâo Paulo. 33 (1): p. 41-46. 2003.

59. GOVERNMENT OF MINAS GERAIS, EDUCATION. Liçôes de Minas: **Merenda - Food is also learned at school**. Minas Gerais: Government of Minas Gerais. p. 63-72. 1999.

60. HARRISON, R.L.; WONG, T. An oral health promotion program for an urban minority population of preschool children. **Community Dent. Oral Epidemiol**. Copenhagen. 31(5): p.392-399. 2003.

61. HAYDT, R. C. C. **Atividades lùdicas na educaçâo da criança / Subsidios prâticos para o trâbalo na pré-escola e nas séries iniciais do 1° grau**. 7ª edition. Sâo Paulo: Editora Âtica. p. 7-15. 1998.

62. HERZLICH, C. The problem of social representation and its usefulness in the field of disease. **Physis Revista de Saùde Coletiva**. 1(2):23-36. 1991.

63. HILL, K. B. et al. Developing a dental health education program (DHE). **Dent. Health.**

London. 40 (4): p. 3-7. 2001.

64. HOLLOWAY, P. J.; ELLWOOD, R. P. The prevalence causes and cosmetic importance of dental fluorosis in the United Kingdom: a review. **Community Dent Health**. 14: 148-55. 1997.

65. KANEGANE, K. et al.Anxiety to dental treatment in emergency care.**Rev. Saùde Pùblica**. [online]. dec. 2003, vol.37, no.6 [cited 22 January 2006], p.786- 792.Disponible naWorldWideWeb:<http://www.scielo.br/scielo.php?script=sci_arttext&pid=S0034 89102003000600015&lng=en&nrm=iso>. ISSN 0034-8910. 2003.

66. KHISHIMOTO, T. M. **O jogo e a educaçâo infantil**. Sâo Paulo: Livraria Pioneira Editora. p. 1-11; 19-24; 39-46. 1994.

67. KOIVISTO, U. K.; SJODÉN, P. O. Reasons for rejection of food items in swedish families with children aged 2-17. **Appetite**. 26: 89-103. 1996.

68. LASCALA, N. T.; MOUSSALI, N. H. Oral Hygiene. In: LASCALA, N. T.; MOUSSALI, N. H. **Compêndio Terapèutico Periodontal**. Sâo Paulo: Editora Artes Médicas. p-240-269. 1995.

69. LEVY, S. M. et al. Infants fluoride ingestion from water, supplements and dentifrice. **JADA**. 126: 1625-1632. 1995.

70. LIMA, Y. B. O.; CURY, J. A. Fluoride ingestion by children through water and toothpaste. **Rev. Saùde Pùblica** (online journal), 2001; 36(6). Available at: http://www.fsp.usp.br. 2001.

71. LOUREIRO, C. F. B. A Educaçâo em Saù na Formaçâo do Educador. **Revista Brasileira de Saùde Escolar**. 4 (3). 1996.

72. MACHADO, M. M. **O brinquedo-sucata e a criança** / A importância de brincar - Atividades e materiais. Sâo Paulo: Ediçôes Loyola. p. 31-39; 49-56. 1994.

73. MALUF, A. C. **Brincar; prazer e aprendizado**. Sâo Paulo: Editora Vozes. p. 32. 2003.

74. MARANHAO, D. G. Caring for the link between health and education. **Cad. Pesqui**. [online]. 2000, no. 111 [cited 2006-11-27], pp. 115-133. Available at: <http://www.scielo.br/scielo.php?script=sci_arttext&pid=S0100-15742000000300006&lng=en&nrm=iso>. ISSN 0100-1574. doi: 10.1590/S0100-15742000000300006. 2000.

75. MARANHAO, D. N. M. **Ensinar brincando: aprendizagem pode ser uma grande brincadeira**. 2.ed. Rio de Janeiro: Wac. p.90. 2003.

76. MARCELLINO, N. C. **Estudos do lazer: uma introduçâo**. Campinas: Autores Associados. p.37. 1996.

77. MARTINS, E. M. Constuindo o Valor Saùde Bucal. **Açâo Coletiva**. 2(2): p. 5-9. 1999.

78. MATOS, O. Modern forms of backwardness. **Folha de Sâo Paulo**, Sâo Paulo, September 27, 1998. Primeiro Caderno, Sâo Paulo. p.3. 1998.

79. MASTRANTONIO, S.S.; GARCIA, P.P.N.S. Educational programs in oral health - literature review. BP: **J. Odontopediatr. Odontol. Baby. Curitiba**. 5 (25): p. 215-222. 2002.

80. MEDEIROS JÛNIOR, A. et al. Extramural experience in a public hospital and the promotion of collective oral health. **Rev. Saùde Pùblica**. Sâo Paulo, 39 (2): IsSN 0034-8910. Print version. 2005.

81. MEDRONHO, R. A. et al. **Epidemiology**. Sâo Paulo: Editora Atheneu. ch. 2, 3. p. 15-55. 2002.

82. MENDES, E.V. **The production of knowledge for dental practice in Latin America**. Paper presented at the First Conference of Dental Schools and Faculties in Latin America, Faculty of Medical Sciences, Autonomous University of Santo Domingo, October 12-16, 1980. mimeogr. Apud PRETO, S.M. A odontologia no SUS: o desafio da pràtica integral. 1991. Dissertation (Master's degree in social dentistry). Fluminense Federal University, 1992.

83. MINAYO, M. C. S.; HARTZ, Z. M. A.; BUSS, P. M. Quality of life and health: a necessary debate. **Ciênc. saùde coletiva**. [online]. 2000, vol. 5, no. 1 [cited 2006-11-28], pp. 7-18. Available from: <http://www.scielo.br/scielo.php?script=sci_arttext&pid=S1413-81232000000100002&lng=en&nrm=iso>. ISSN 1413-8123. doi: 10.1590/S1413-81232000000100002. 2000.

84. MONTEIRO, C. A.; CONDE, W. L.; CASTRO, I. R. R. The changing trend in the relationship between schooling and risk of obesity in Brazil. **Cadernos de Saùblica**. 19(1): 67-75. 2003.

85. MOTTA, L. G. et al. Total fluoride and pH of toothpastes on the market in Rio de Janeiro. **RBO**. 59(2): 136-138. 2002.

86. MUNGUBA, M. C. Videogames: learning strategies. **The occupational therapist's vision for the 21st century**. Support for occupational therapists, educators and parents. Fortaleza: University of Fortaleza; 2002.

87. MWANGOSI, I. E. A. T.; MWAKATOBE, K. M.; ASTROM, A. N. K. Sources of oral health

information and teaching materials for primary school teachers in Rungwe district, Tanzania. **Int. Dent. J.. London**. 52 (6): p. 469-474. 2002.

88. NEIRA E. P. H. Brinquedo no hospital. **Rev. Esc. Enfermagem USP**. 3 (24): p. 319-28. 1990.

89. NÓBREGA, F. J. **Distùrbios da nutricçao**. Rio de Janeiro: Livraria e Editora Revinter. p. 14, 42-43, 175-181. 1998.

90. NEW PEDAGOGICAL EDITION FOR THE MODERN SCHOOL. Annual course plan / Methodology and activities. 1st grade. **Health education**. General supervision: Arnaldo Soveral. Curitiba. p. 150- 153, 463-499. 1989.

91. NEW PEDAGOGICAL EDITION FOR THE MODERN SCHOOL. Annual course plan / Methodology and activities. 2nd grade. **Health education**. General supervision: Arnaldo Soveral. Curitiba. p. 115-118, 526-580. 1989.

92. NEW PEDAGOGICAL EDITION FOR THE MODERN SCHOOL. Annual course plan / Methodology and activities. 3rd grade. **Health education**. General supervision: Arnaldo Soveral. Curitiba. p. 93-94, 515-579. 1989.

93. NEW PEDAGOGICAL EDITION FOR THE MODERN SCHOOL. Annual course plan / Methodology and activities. 4th grade. **Health education**. General supervision: Arnaldo Soveral. Curitiba. p. 85-93, 547-618. 1989.

94. NÓVOA, A. Teacher training and the teaching profession. In: NÓVOA, A. (Org.). **Os professores e sua formaçâo**. Lisbon: Publicaçôes Dom Quixote - Instituto de Inovaçâo Educacional. p. 97-121. 1997.

95. OAKLANDER, V. **Discovering children: the gestalt approach with children and adolescents**. Translated by George Schlesinger. Sâo Paulo: Summus. p. 17-46; 183-190; 308313. 1980.

96. OKESON, J. P. **Treatment of temporomandibular disorders and occlusion**. 4ª edition. São Paulo: Artes Médicas. p. 1-100. 2000.

97. WORLD HEALTH ORGANIZATION, O. M. S. Health-promoting school: Healthy environment and better health for future generations. Communication for health n. 13.

Pan American Sanitary Department, Regional Department of the O. M. S. Translation: Renata Ferreira e Ferreira. Washington, D.C. Printed version. p. 1-19. 1998.

98. PETTRY, P. C.; PRETTO. S. M. Education and motivation in oral health. In KRIGER, L. **Oral health promotion: ABOPREV**. Sâo Paulo : Artes Médicas. p. 364-370. 1997.

99. PHILIPPI, S. T. et al . Adapted food pyramid: a guide for a right food choice. **Rev. Nutr, Campinas**, v. 12, n. 1, 1999. Available from: http://www.scielo.br/scielo.php?script=sci_arttext&pid=S1415-52731999000100006&lng=en&nrm=iso>. Accessed on: 08 Nov 2006. doi: 10.1590/S1415-52731999000100006. 1999.

100. PILON, A. F. The development of health education: an updating of concepts. **Rev. Saùde Pùblica**. [online]. 1986, vol. 20, no. 5 [cited 2006-11-28], pp. 391-396. Available from: <http://www.scielo.br/scielo.php?script=sci_arttext&pid=S0034-89101986000500009&lng=en&nrm=iso>. ISSN 0034-8910. doi: 10.1590/S0034-89101986000500009. 1986.

101. PINTO, M. Childhood as a social construction. In: SARMENTO, Jacinto (org). **Children: contexts and identities**. Minho-Portugal: Centro de Estudos da Criança. p. 31-73. 1997.

102. PIOTTO, D. C. et al. Promoting quality and evaluation in early childhood education: an experience. **Cadernos de Pesquisa**. Sâo Paulo. 1 (105): p. 52-77. 1998.

103. POLETTO, R. C. Children's playfulness and its relationship with the family context. **Psicologia em Estudo. Maringâ**. 10(1): p. 67-75. 2005.

104. PORTILLO, J. A. C.; PAES, A M. C. Self-perception of oral health-related quality of life. **Rev Bras. de Odont. em Saùde Coletiva**. 1 (1): p.75-88. 2000.

105. RAMOS, M.; STEIN, L. M. Development of infant eating behavior. **Jornal de Pediatria**. 76(3): 229-237. 2000.

106. REGO, T. C. Culture becomes part of human nature.In: . **Vygotsky: a historical-cultural perspective of education**. 11ª ed. Petrópolis: Vozes. p.37-83. 2001.

107. RIZZI, L.; HAYDT, R. C. C. **Atividades lùdicas na educaçâo da criança: subsidios prâticos para o trabalho na pré-escola e nas séries iniciais do 1° grau.** 7th edition. Sâo Paulo: Editora Atica. p. 7-15. 1998.

108. ROCHA, C.M.V. Educaçâo em saùde: breve histórico e perspectivas. In: BRAZIL. Ministry of Health. **Coletânea educaçâo, saùde e educaçâo em saùde**. Brasilia, DF, 1989.

109. ROCHA, M. S. P. M. L. **Nâo brinco mais: a (des)construção do brincar no cotidiano educacional**. Ijui: Unijui. p. 66. 2000.

110. RODRIGUES, M. **O desenvolvimento do pré-escolar e o jogo**. Sâo Paulo: Editora icone. p. 45-61. 1992.

111. ROSSETTI, H. **Saúde para a Odontologia** - Hugo Rossetti / Translation: Sônia Cristina Lima Chaves / Review: Carla Cristina Luz Leal, Marilda Ivanov. 2nd ed. Sâo Paulo: Editora Santos. 146 p. 1999.

112. ROUQUAYROL, M. Z. **Epidemiology & Health**. Epidemiology, Natural History and Disease Prevention. In: Rouquayrol, M. Z. 4th edition. Rio de Janeiro: MEDSI. p. 7-22. 1993.

113. RUFINO NETTO, A. Qualidade de Vida: Compromisso Histórico da Epidemiologia.

Quality of life: epidemiology's historical commitment. In MFL Lima e Costa & RP Sousa (eds.). Coopmed/Abrasco. Belo Horizonte. p. 11-18. 1994.

114. SALGADO, R. G.; PEREIRA, R. M. R.; SOUZA, S. J. Through the screen, through the window: theoretical and practical questions about childhood and television. **Cad. Cedes**. Campinas. 25(65): 9-24. 2005.

115. SALIBA, N. A. et al. Oral health education program: the experience of the Araçatuba School of Dentistry -UNESP. **Rev. Odontologia Clin.-Cientif**. Recife, 2 (3): 197200. 2003.

116. SANTOS, P.A. et al. Education and motivation: impact of different methods on children's learning. JBP: 46 Garcia et al. **Revista de Odontologia da UNESP J.**

Pediatric Dentistry Baby. Curitiba. 5 (26): p. 310-315. 2002a

117. SANTOS, P. A. Evaluation of the knowledge of elementary school teachers from private schools about oral health. **Rev. Odontol. UNESP**, Sâo Paulo. 31(2): p.205-214. 2002b.

118. SANTOS, S. M. P. **Brinquedo e infância: um guia para pais e educadores em creche**. Petrópolis: Vozes. p.7. 1999.

119. SECRETARIAT OF HEALTH. Resolution SS-95, of 06/27/2000. **Recommendations on the use of fluoride dentifrices within the scope of the SUS/SP as a function of the risk of dental caries**. (online), available at: http://www.saude.sp.gov.br. 2000.

120. SERRA, M. C.; CURY, J. A. Fluoride kinetics in saliva after the use of fluoridated dentifrices and mouthwashes. **Rev. Assoc. Paul. Cirur. Dent**. 46(5): 875-878. 1992.

121. SICHIERI, R.; CASTRO, J. F. G.; MOURA, A. S. Factors associated with the food consumption pattern of the urban Brazilian population. **Cadernos de Saùblica**. 19(1): 57-53. 2003.

122. SILVA, M. B. C. **Storytelling / An art without age**. 7ª edition. Sâo Paulo: Editora Atica. p. 7-12. 1997.

123. SILVA, M. F. A. **Systemic Fluoride: Basic, toxicological and clinical aspects**. In: KRIGER, L. Promoçâo de Saúde Bucal: ABOPREV. 2nd edition. Sâo Paulo: Artes Médicas. p.141-166. 1999.

124. SOUZA, L. J. E. X.; RODRIGUES A. K. C.; BARROSO, M. G. T. A familia vivenciar o acidente doméstico: relato de experiência. **Rev Latino-Am.Enferm**. 8:83-9. 2000.

125. TOJO, R. et al. Eating habits of preschool and school-age children: health risks and strategies for intervention. **Summary of the 37th Nestlé Nutrition Seminar**. 11-13.

126. TORRIANI, D. D. Dental Caries. In: Busato, A. L. S. **Dentistica / Restorations in posterior teeth**. Sâo Paulo: Artes Médicas Publishing House. Chap.1. p. 1-22. 1996.

127. VALENÇA, A. M. G. **Health education in the training of dental surgeons: from necessity to participatory practice**. Monograph (Specialization in Public Health Education). Rio de Janeiro, Fluminense Federal University. 1992.

128. VALLA, V.V. Education, health and citizenship: scientific research and popular advice. **Cadernos de saùblica**. Rio de Janeiro. 1 (8): p. 30-40. 1982.

129. VENTURA D. V. R. **Participatory action as an educational practice in leprosy control**. In: Brasil. Ministry of Health. Coletânea educaçâo, saù e educaçâo em saù. Brasilia, DF, 1989.

130. VIEIRA, L. J. E. S. et al. Play in the prevention of accidents in children from 4 to 6 years old. **RBPS**. 18 (2) : 78-84. 2005.

131. VITOLO, M. R. **Nutriçao da gestação à adolescência**. Rio de Janeiro: Reichmann & Autores Editores. p. 144-151. 2003.

132. VYGOTSKY, L.S. **The social formation of the mind**. Sâo Paulo, SP: Livraria Martins Fontes. p. 16. 1988.

133. WEISS, L. **Brinquedos & Engenhocas / Playful activities with scrap**. Sâo Paulo: Editora Scipione. p. 19-28. 1997.

134. WELSH, S., DAVIS, C., SHAW, A. Development of the food guide pyramid. **Nutrition Today**, Annapolis. 27(6): p.12-23. 1992b.

ANNEXES

ANNEX I

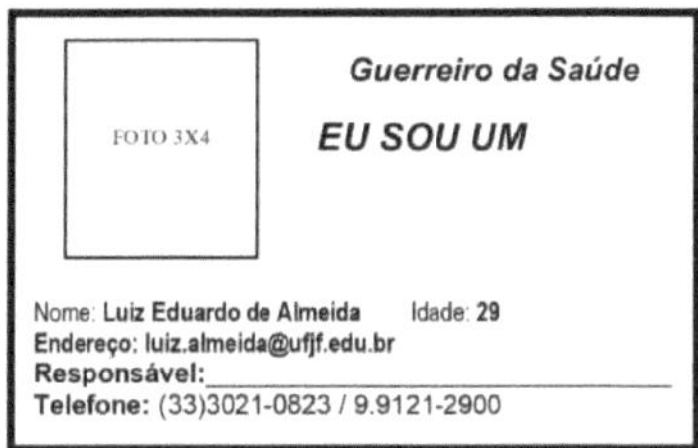

FOTO 3X4

Guerreiro da Saúde

EU SOU UM

Nome: Luiz Eduardo de Almeida Idade: 29
Endereço: luiz.almeida@ufjf.edu.br
Responsável:____________________
Telefone: (33)3021-0823 / 9.9121-2900

ANNEX II

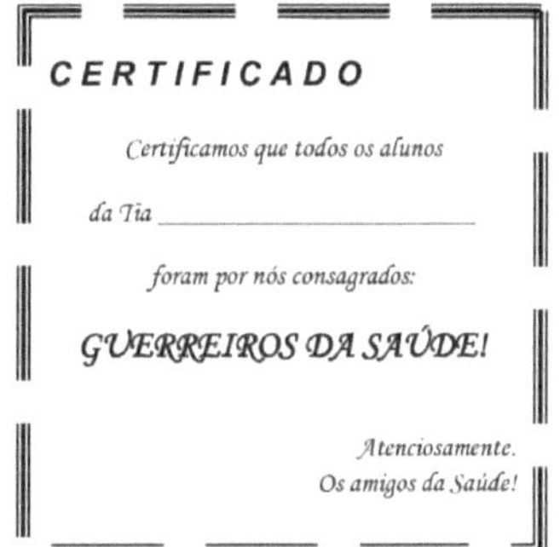

CERTIFICADO

Certificamos que todos os alunos

da Tia ____________________

foram por nós consagrados:

GUERREIROS DA SAÚDE!

Atenciosamente.
Os amigos da Saúde!

Annex III

Warning letter

Parents and/or guardians, this letter informs you that your child may be part of a study which has the following descriptions:

1. Main objective: to verify the effect of a motivational, self-instruction method on oral and general health knowledge. The specific objectives are: to make children carriers of knowledge, as well as to make them aware of the importance of prevention education; to propose simple and low-cost educational and motivational strategies; to provide schoolchildren with a better level of knowledge about general and oral health, combining education with pleasure; to aim for a better relationship between schoolchildren and health professionals; to demystify beliefs, attitudes and inadequate behavior in relation to health. However, the school will be differentiated by its characteristics, being considered a "Health Promoting School".

3. **Justification/Benefits:** This work is justified by the great need to introduce in Brazil, especially in poor communities, the awareness of the population of the importance of preventive procedures in relation to health, not only physical, but also mental. Through the introduction of strategies related to general and oral health, the aim is to teach the group served about the possibility of avoiding illnesses by changing inappropriate habits, making this learner a carrier of health knowledge.

4. **Procedures:** Two questionnaires will be administered, one to the family and the other to the children. Health education will be developed through lectures and recreational activities. The questionnaires will be administered at the beginning, middle and end of the project for further data analysis, where learning, apprehension and the sharing of information by the children will be assessed.

5. **Expected risks:** The evaluations will be risk-free for those assisted.

6. **Compensation, expenses and reimbursement:** under no circumstances will the research participants be paid or compensated for their participation and they will not incur any expenses in carrying out the study.

7. **Guaranteed access:** At any stage of the study, parents or guardians will have access to the professionals and academics responsible for the research to clarify any doubts.

8. **Withdrawal from the study:** Parents or guardians may request that their child withdraw from the study at any time, without any harm to them.

9. **Right to Confidentiality:** The information obtained during the evaluations will be kept completely confidential, but may be used for statistical or scientific purposes, and the identification of any child will not be disclosed.

10. **Right of access to results:** Parents or guardians will have the right to access the results of the survey at any time, even if they are only partial.

11. **Obligations** of **the volunteer:** Volunteers must provide the researcher with correct information.

12. **Personal harm:** The procedures that will be carried out are not expected to cause any harm to children.

13. **Free and Informed Consent:**

I, Mr. ____, bearer of

ID No., residing at

and telephone number ____________I, the minor's guardian, certify that, having read the previous information and having been sufficiently informed by the guardians about all the items, I am in full agreement with the carrying out of the study, authorizing the minor to participate ________________________in the study as a volunteer.

This informed consent form will be issued in two copies, one of which will remain with me and the other with the researcher in charge.

____ of of

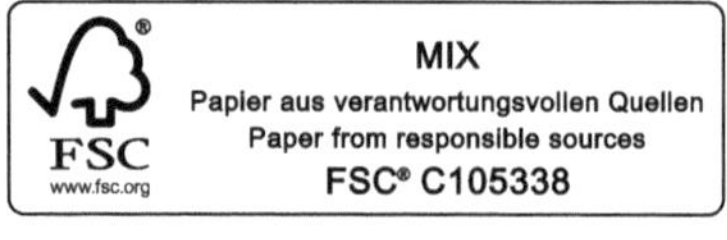

Printed by Books on Demand GmbH, Norderstedt / Germany